## An Atlas of Investigation and Management
# CONNECTIVE TISSUE DISEASES

An Atlas of Investigation and Management

# CONNECTIVE TISSUE DISEASES

**Caroline Gordon, MD FRCP**

Professor and Consultant in Rheumatology
School of Immunity and Infection
College of Medical and Dental Sciences
The Medical School, University of Birmingham
Birmingham, UK

**Wolfgang L Gross, MD PhD**

Medical Director & Chairman
Department of Rheumatology
University of Luebeck & Clinic for Rheumatology, Bad Bramstedt
Luebeck, Germany

**CLINICAL PUBLISHING**

OXFORD

**Clinical Publishing**
an imprint of Atlas Medical Publishing Ltd
Oxford Centre for Innovation
Mill Street, Oxford OX2 0JX, UK

Tel: +44 1865 811116
Fax: +44 1865 251550
Email: info@clinicalpublishing.co.uk
Web: www.clinicalpublishing.co.uk

**Distributed in USA and Canada by:**
Clinical Publishing
30 Amberwood Parkway
Ashland, OH 44805, USA

Tel: 800-247-6553 (toll free within US and Canada)
Fax: 419-281-6883
Email: order@bookmasters.com

**Distributed in UK and Rest of World by:**
Marston Book Services Ltd
PO Box 269
Abingdon
Oxon OX14 4YN, UK

Tel: +44 1235 465500
Fax: +44 1235 465555
Email: trade.orders@marston.co.uk

A catalogue record of this book is available from the British Library

ISBN print     978 1 84692 074 5
ISBN e-book  978 1 84692 634 1

**The publisher makes no representation, express or implied, that the dosages in this book are correct. Readers must therefore always check the product information and clinical procedures with the most up-to-date published product information and data sheets provided by the manufacturers and the most recent codes of conduct and safety regulations. The authors and the publisher do not accept any liability for any errors in the text or for the misuse or misapplication of material in this work.**

**Clinical Publishing and Atlas Medical Publishing Ltd bear no responsibility for the persistence or accuracy of URLs for external or third-party internet websites referred to in this publication, and do not guarantee that any content on such websites is, or will remain, accurate or appropriate.**

Colour reproduction by Tenon & Polert Colour Scanning Ltd, Hong Kong
Printed by Marston Book Services Ltd, Abingdon, Oxon, UK

# Contents

# Preface

Patients that present with a connective tissue disease are often a challenge to diagnose and treat. A connective tissue disease is a disorder in which the tissues of the body consisting of the cells and the matrix which holds them together are disrupted. This atlas will describe the multi-system conditions that result from inflammatory and immune-mediated disorders that can affect all the tissues of the body and their management, including presentation, investigation, differential diagnosis and treatment. Systemic lupus erythematosus, Sjögren's syndrome, anti-phospholipid syndrome, idiopathic inflammatory myopathies, systemic sclerosis and the primary systemic vasculitides will be discussed in detail. These diseases are multifactorial conditions associated with a complex genetic predisposition and various, not well-understood, environmental triggers that induce inflammatory and immune-mediated responses directed against components of the person's own body. As a result this group of diseases is known also as the systemic autoimmune diseases. This atlas will not discuss the inherited connective disorders due to genetic mutations that affect collagen (Ehlers–Danlos syndrome) and other connective tissue proteins, such as fibrillin-1 in Marfan's syndrome.

Patients with a systemic autoimmune connective tissue disease can present with clinical symptoms and signs in one or more often, several, systems of the body. Some of these diseases affect people of certain ages and gender more often than others, including children, but this atlas will focus on the management of adult patients. These diseases are more common than is generally realized, cannot be cured, are associated with considerable morbidity and still cause significant mortality. Appropriate investigations are critical to making the correct diagnosis so that treatment can be tailored to the patient's condition. It is important not only to recognize and treat the current disease activity, but also to prevent death and the development of chronic damage due to complications of the disease and the immunosuppressive drugs used to treat it. Treatment usually includes immunosuppressive therapy and other drugs depending on the effects of the disease on specific organs of the body. Principles of drug treatment will be discussed in this atlas, but the final choice of drug and exact dosages to be used will depend on the details of the patient's condition and should be planned by a physician with relevant experience of these conditions and responsible for the management of the patient.

Due to the variable severity of these diseases and their multisystem nature that may deteriorate in pregnancy, patients with an autoimmune connective tissue disease may present to general practioners, general physicians or internal medicine specialists, obstetricians, intensive care or any medical or surgical specialist. The majority of patients with these conditions are cared for long term by dermatologists, rheumatologists, and/or nephrologists, as it is the skin, joints and kidneys that are most often involved. However it should be noted that many patients develop cardio-respiratory or infectious complications, including accelerated atherosclerosis, due to the disease and/or its treatment. Multidisciplinary care is important and should involve the full range of allied health professionals, as well as the relevant clinical specialists depending on the organs and systems involved.

Caroline Gordon
Wolfgang L Gross

# Editors and contributors

## Editors

**Caroline Gordon, MD FRCP**
Professor and Consultant in Rheumatology
School of Immunity and Infection
College of Medical and Dental Services
The Medical School, University of Birmingham
Birmingham, UK

**Wolfgang L Gross, MD PhD**
Medical Director & Chairman
Department of Rheumatology
University of Luebeck & Clinic for Rheumatology,
    Bad Bramstedt
Luebeck, Germany

## Contributors

**Philip Clements, MD MPH**
Professor of Medicine
Division of Rheumatology
David Geffen School of Medicine at UCLA
Los Angeles, CA, USA

**Daniel E Furst, MD**
Carl M Pearson Professor of Rheumatology
Director of Rheumatology Therapeutic Research
University of California in Los Angeles
Los Angeles, CA, USA

**Ariane L Herrick, MD FRCP**
Professor of Rheumatology
The University of Manchester
Manchester Academic Health Science Centre
Salford Royal Hospital
Salford, UK

**Julia U Holle, MD**
Department of Rheumatology
University of Lübeck and Klinikum Bad Bramstedt
Bad Bramstedt, Germany

**Iona Meryon, MBChB MRCP**
Department of Rheumatology
Chelsea and Westminster Hospital NHS Foundation Trust
London, UK

**Frank Moosig, MD PhD**
University Hospital of Schleswig-Holstein and Klinikum
    Bad Bramstedt
Bad Bramstedt, Germany

# Abbreviations

5-FDG 5-fluorodeoxyglucose
AAV ANCA-associated vasculitides
ACEI angiotensin-converting enzyme inhibitor
ACR American College of Rheumatology
ALT alanine transferase
AMA anti-mitochondrial antibody
ANA anti-nuclear antibody
ANCA anti-neutrophil cytoplasmic antibody
APS anti-phospholipid syndrome
ARB angiotensin-receptor blocker
ARDS acute respiratory distress syndrome
AST aspartate transaminase
AZA azathioprine
BMD bone mineral density
BVAS Birmingham Vasculitis Activity Score
cANCA cytoplasmic ANCA
CAP community acquired pneumonia
CCB calcium-channel blocker
CHCC Chapel Hill Consensus Conference
CK creatine kinase
CK-MB creatine kinase MB isoenzyme
CLA cutanous (isolated) leukocytoclastic angiitis
CMV cytomegalovirus
CNS central nervous system
CRP C-reactive protein
CSS Churg–Strauss syndrome
CT computed tomography
CV cryoglobulinaemic vasculitis
CYC cyclophosphamide
DEXA dual energy X-ray absorptiometry
DILS diffuse infiltrative lymphocytosis syndrome
DM dermatomyositis
(ds)DNA (double-stranded) deoxyribonucleic acid
DVT deep vein thrombosis
EBV Epstein–Barr virus

ECG electrocardiogram
EGD oesophago-gastroduodenostomy
EMG electromyography
ENA extractable nuclear antigen
ENT ear, nose, and throat
ERA endothelin receptor antagonist
ESR erythrocyte sedimentation rate
FVC forced vital capacity
GC glucocorticoids
GCA giant cell arteritis
GERD gastro-oesophageal reflux disease
GI gastrointestinal
HCQ hydroxychloroquine
HCV hepatitis C-associated cryglobulinaemic vasculitis
HDU high dependency unit
HIV human immunodeficiency virus
HRCT high resolution computed tomography
HSP Henoch–Schönlein purpura
HTLV human T-lymphotrophic virus
IBM inclusion body myositis
IFN interferon
Ig immunoglobulin
IIM idiopathic inflammatory myopathy
IL interleukin
ILD interstitial lung disease
INR international normalized ratio
ITP immune thrombocytopaenic purpura
IVIG intravenous immunoglobulin
KD Kawasaki's disease
LDH lactate dehydrogenase
MAA myositis-associated autoantibody
MALT mucosa-associated lymphoid tissue
MI myocardial infarction
MMF mycophenolate mofetil
MPA microscopic polyangiitis

MPO myeloperoxidase
MR magnetic resonance
MRC Medical Research Council
MS multiple sclerosis
MSA myositis-specific autoantibody
MTX methotrexate
NHL non-Hodgkin's lymphoma
NIH National Institutes of Health
NISP nonspecific interstitial pneumonitis
NSAID nonsteroidal anti-inflammatory drug
NTG nitroglycerin
PAH pulmonary arterial hypertension
PAN polyarteritis nodosa
PBC primary biliary cirrhosis
PCR polymerase chain reaction
PDE-5 phosphodiesterase-5
PET positron emission tomography
PM polymyositis
PMR polymyalgia rheumatica
PPI proton-pump inhibitor
PR3 proteinase 3
PSV primary systemic vasculitides

PVD pulmonary vascular disease
RCT randomized controlled trial
RF rheumatoid factor
RV rheumatoid vasculitis
RVSP right ventricular systolic pressure
SGOT serum glutamic oxaloacetic transaminase
SGPT serum glutamic pyruvic transaminase
SIBO small intestinal bacterial overgrowth
SLAM systemic lupus activity measure
SLE systemic lupus erythematosus
SPARC secreted protein, acidic and rich in cysteine
SRC scleroderma renal crisis
SS Sjögren's syndrome
SSc systemic sclerosis
STIR short tau inversion recovery
TA Takayasu's arteritis
TGF tumour growth factor
TIA transient ischaemic attack
TNF tumour necrosis factor
ULN upper limit of normal
UV ultraviolet
WG Wegener's granulomatosis

# Chapter 1

# General approach to the assessment of patients with a suspected connective tissue disease

*Ariane L Herrick*

## Introduction

Connective tissue diseases including the vasculitides can be difficult to diagnose, yet early diagnosis is essential in order to initiate effective treatment as soon as possible, and thereby prevent/minimize tissue injury. Therefore, the key point is to be able to recognize the clinical features which prompt the question 'Could this patient have a connective tissue disease or vasculitis?' Early treatment can be lifesaving, as exemplified by Scenarios 1 and 2.

### Scenario 1

A 55-year-old male was admitted with profound lethargy and swollen wrists, knees, and ankles, and recent haemoptysis (he was a heavy smoker). On examination he was pale, with synovitis of his wrists and knees (with small knee effusions) and pitting oedema of both ankles. He was anaemic with a haemoglobin of 99 g/l (normocytic), erythrocyte sedimentation rate (ESR) was very high at 113 mm/h. Plasma biochemistry showed impaired renal function (urea 14.8 mmol/l, creatinine 190 µmol/l) with a low albumin at 30 g/l. Chest X-ray showed a cavitating lesion of the left upper zone. The following day his creatinine had risen to 250 µmol/l. No dipstick testing of urine had been performed on admission – 1 day later this showed blood and protein.

The medical registrar initially queried a paraneoplastic syndrome with some dehydration. However, when the dipstick and repeat renal function results were seen the following day, the working diagnosis was revised to a connective tissue disease, possibly vasculitis. The renal team performed an urgent renal biopsy and intravenous methylprednisolone was commenced. Renal biopsy showed necrotizing glomerulonephritis, and intravenous cyclophosphamide was added to the drug regime. Initially

the renal function deteriorated further but 2 weeks later began to improve. Immunology testing was positive for anti-neutrophil cytoplasmic antibody (cytoplasmic pattern, cANCA), consistent with the clinical impression of Wegener's granulomatosis, which had been made on the basis of a cavitating lung lesion, renal vasculitis, inflammatory arthritis, and systemic inflammation.

### Scenario 2

A 43-year-old female was admitted with a 3-day history of breathlessness and general malaise. On examination, her temperature was 38°C, she had basal crackles, and poor air entry. Haemoglobin was 109 g/l, white blood cell count 4.9 × 10⁹/l, platelets 120 × 10⁹/l. ESR was 45 mm/h. Chest X-ray showed widespread interstitial shadowing.

The working diagnosis was of community acquired pneumonia (CAP). However, despite antibiotic therapy her condition deteriorated rapidly with falling $PO_2$ and she was transferred to the high dependency unit (HDU). The medical registrar who assessed the patient in the HDU noted that she had felt tired for around 2 months, had been suffering from mouth ulcers, and had recently begun experiencing Raynaud's phenomenon. An autoimmune screen showed that she was strongly anti-nuclear antibody (ANA) positive (1/10,000) with a high titre of anti-double-stranded deoxyribonucleic acid (dsDNA) antibodies (155 U/ml, reference range 0–7).

The diagnosis was revised to pneumonitis secondary to systemic lupus erythematosus (SLE), and she was treated with intravenous methylprednisolone, followed later by oral prednisolone. After commencing steroids her clinical condition improved and the shadowing on chest X-ray resolved.

### Discussion of Scenarios 1 and 2

Although Scenarios 1 and 2 describe patients with recent onset, fulminating illness, most patients with connective tissue disease (including vasculitis) do not present with immediately life-threatening illnesses, but have been unwell for some time before a diagnosis is made. Clinical features are often nonspecific, especially early in the disease. Connective tissue disease should always be suspected in a patient who presents with multisystem inflammatory disease.

The first step is to establish the diagnosis, recognizing that many patients have overlapping features between different connective tissue diseases/vasculitides. Once a diagnosis is made, the emphasis of assessment changes. It then concentrates on assessment of activity and severity, and identification of new internal organ involvement. Assessment of activity and severity of the different connective tissue diseases is discussed mainly in the disease-based chapters. Patients with connective tissue disease usually need to be under long-term specialist review, the main purpose of this being to recognize changes in disease activity and severity necessitating changes in management.

## History-taking and the assessment of symptoms

The key point is to take a full history as most tissues/organs can be affected in patients with connective tissue disease.

### Presenting complaint

This may be virtually anything, examples being lethargy, breathlessness, heartburn, abdominal pain, paraesthesia, and rash.

### Systemic enquiry
#### General

Common symptoms are tiredness and weight loss. Patients may also report fever, but it must be remembered that fever in patients with suspected or established connective tissue disease may be due to infection, to which they may be predisposed as a result of either the underlying disease or its treatment. For example, infection is a major contributor to mortality in patients with SLE, who are often complement deficient and who are frequently treated with steroids and/or immunosuppressant drugs. These symptoms – tiredness, weight loss, and fever – are all nonspecific and occur in malignancy and infection as well as in connective tissue disease (*Table 1.1*). To complicate matters further, there are associations between certain autoimmune diseases and malignancy; therefore, even in the patient with established connective tissue disease, the clinician always needs to be alert to the development of concomitant disease.

### Skin and mucous membranes

Rashes occur in several of the connective tissue diseases, as described more fully under 'Examination'. If a patient complains of a rash, always ask if it is photosensitive: classically the 'butterfly' rash of SLE is photosensitive. Cutaneous ulcers occur especially in systemic sclerosis (SSc), when usually the fingers or toes are affected (see below), and in the vasculitides. Hair loss (patchy or diffuse) occurs commonly in SLE (**1.1**). Mouth ulcers (**1.2**) occur commonly in SLE and Behçet's syndrome (in which genital ulcers also occur). Oral dryness is one of the main symptoms of Sjögren's syndrome. Other features are described in *Table 1.2* and below under 'Examination'.

---

**Table 1.1 Nonspecific manifestations of connective tissue disease or vasculitis**

| Manifestations (may occur separately or in any combination) | Differential diagnoses to be considered |
| --- | --- |
| Fatigue/tiredness/malaise | Infection |
| Fever | Connective tissue disease |
| Weight loss | Vasculitis |
| Enlarged lymph nodes | Malignancy (including lymphoma) |

**Table 1.2 Typical skin manifestations in connective tissue disease**

*SLE*

Photosensitive ('butterfly') rash

Alopecia

Mouth ulcers

*APS*

Livido reticularis

*Systemic sclerosis*

Scleroderma

Digital pitting/ulceration

Telangiectases

Calcinosis

*Dermatomyositis*

Facial rash ('heliotrope') with periorbital oedema

Gottron's papules

Periungal erythema

*Vasculitis*

Splinter haemorrhages and nailfold infarcts

Purpura

Oral and genital ulcers in Behçet's syndrome

Cutaneous ulcers

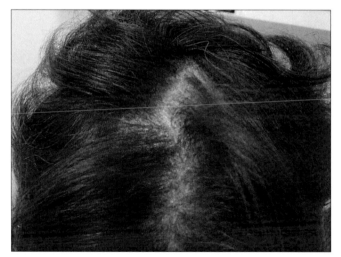

**1.1** Diffuse alopecia in a patient with systemic lupus erythematosus.

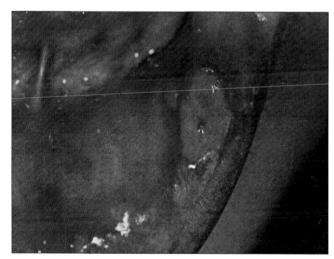

**1.2** Aphthous mouth ulcer. (Courtesy of Dr. M. Pemberton.)

### Raynaud's phenomenon

This occurs commonly in connective tissue disease, especially in SSc, in which it is rare not to have Raynaud's. The classic episodic colour changes of the fingers (white, then blue/purple, then red) occur typically in response to cold exposure or to stress (**1.3**). In Scenario 2, the point of interest about the Raynaud's phenomenon was that it had commenced only recently: patients with primary (idiopathic) Raynaud's phenomenon typically develop this in their teens or early 20s. When Raynaud's phenomenon occurs in patients with underlying connective tissue disease

it can progress to irreversible tissue injury with ulceration, scarring, or gangrene. Worrying features in the history are a persistent fingertip discoloration and the development of digital ulceration.

### Musculoskeletal

Involvement of the musculoskeletal system is common (*Table 1.3*). Patients with connective tissue disease often have arthralgia. They may also develop an inflammatory arthritis with joint pain, swelling, and stiffness. Proximal

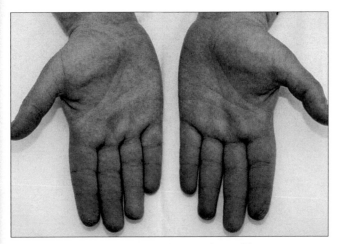

**1.3** Raynaud's phenomenon in a patient with undifferentiated connective tissue disease: several of the digits are cyanosed.

muscle pain and weakness occur in inflammatory muscle disease: the patient has difficulty getting out of bed or out of a chair, especially first thing in the morning. Proximal muscle weakness may also be a side-effect of chronic use of corticosteroids.

*Cardiorespiratory*
A number of different forms of heart or lung involvement may occur including pulmonary fibrosis, pneumonia, pulmonary embolism (especially in those with anti-phospholipid syndrome [APS]), pericardial effusion, valvular heart disease or (especially in SSc) arrhythmia (*Table 1.4*). Therefore, all cardiorespiratory symptoms should be asked about if not volunteered, including breathlessness, chest pain, and oedema. Patients with connective tissue disease, especially SLE, are at increased

---

**Table 1.3 Musculoskeletal symptoms and signs in connective tissue disease or vasculitis**

| *Joints* | *Muscles* |
|---|---|
| Pain (arthralgia) | Pain (myalgia) |
| Early morning stiffness | Early morning stiffness |
| Joint line tenderness | Proximal muscle tenderness |
| Joint swelling (synovial hypertrophy +/- effusion) | Proximal muscle weakness |
| Reduced range of movement | |

---

**Table 1.4 Some examples of cardiorespiratory manifestations of connective tissue disease or vasculitis**

| *Cardiac manifestations* | *Pulmonary manifestations* |
|---|---|
| Pericarditis | Pleurisy |
| Pericardial effusion | Pleural effusion |
| Angina | Pulmonary embolism |
| Arrhythmias | Pneumonitis |
| Cardiac failure | Lung fibrosis |
| Valvular heart disease | Haemoptysis |

---

**Table 1.5 Some examples of gastrointestinal symptoms of connective tissue disease or vasculitis by region**

| *Upper gastrointestinal tract* | *Lower gastrointestinal tract* |
|---|---|
| Mucosal ulceration | Abdominal pain |
| Acid reflux | Change in bowel habit |
| Dysphagia | Blood loss in stools |

risk of coronary artery disease and should therefore be specifically asked about symptoms.

### Gastrointestinal

Gastrointestinal (GI) features are often not recognized as being due to connective tissue disease or vasculitis (*Table 1.5*). Swallowing difficulty, often with reflux symptoms, is very common in patients with SSc who may experience a wide range of GI symptoms including alteration in bowel habit: diarrhoea may reflect bacterial overgrowth, and constipation, colonic dysmotility. Abdominal pain can (rarely) be caused by mesenteric ischaemia, which can occur in patients with vasculitis.

### Renal

Ankle swelling has a long differential diagnosis but includes nephrotic syndrome, which can occur for example in SLE.

### Neuropsychiatric

As with the other organ systems, almost any symptom can occur in patients with connective tissue disease. SLE can be associated with involvement of peripheral, central, and autonomic nervous systems as well as with cognitive impairment and psychiatric disturbance (*Table 1.6*). An important point is that neuropsychiatric features can occur not only as a primary manifestation of connective tissue disease but also indirectly: for example, as a result of hypertension, uraemia, infection, coagulation problems (as in APS), or as a result of drug treatment, especially with corticosteroids. Paraesthesia is a common feature in patients with connective tissue disease and can have many causes, for example, peripheral neuropathy or (in the upper limb) carpal tunnel syndrome. Many patients with connective tissue diseases, as with other chronic diseases, become depressed.

### Eyes

The commonest symptom is of dry, gritty eyes, occurring in patients with Sjögren's syndrome. Eye dryness can be confirmed using Schirmer's tear test (**1.4**).

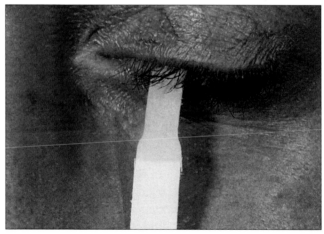

**1.4** Schirmer's test. In this case showing satisfactory wetting of the filter paper.

| Table 1.6 Some examples of neuropsychiatric manifestations of connective tissue disease or vasculitis by region | |
| --- | --- |
| *Region* | *Manifestations* |
| Peripheral nervous system | Paraesthesia in distribution of a nerve, e.g. median nerve |
| | Weakness in distribution of a nerve, e.g. ulnar nerve |
| Central nervous system | Psychosis |
| | Seizures |
| | Hemiplegic stroke |
| | Transverse myelitis |
| Autonomic nervous system | Postural hypotension |

### Drug history

A detailed drug history is important because:

- Connective tissue disease (especially SLE and small vessel vasculitis) can be a side-effect of certain drugs. For example, minocycline can cause SLE or vasculitis.
- Drugs used in the treatment of connective tissue disease may cause side-effects which are difficult to distinguish from active disease. For example, methotrexate may cause pneumonitis and several immunosuppressants may cause pancytopenia.

Two common clinical dilemmas are:

1 A patient with dermatomyositis complains of increasing muscle weakness. Is this active disease despite steroids (necessitating an increase in dosage) or is it steroid-related myopathy (necessitating a reduction in dosage)?
2 A patient with SLE on azathioprine (or another imunosuppressant) develops pancytopenia. Is this active SLE (necessitating an increase in dosage) or is it azathioprine-related bone marrow toxicity (necessitating a reduction in dosage)?

In both these examples, a careful history and examination, backed up by appropriate investigations, should indicate whether the drug treatment should be increased or reduced.

### Family history

There is likely to be a genetic component to most of the connective tissue diseases, although the absolute risk to family members is small. For example, although the single most important risk factor for SSc is a positive family history, the risk for each family member is less than 1%. Perhaps more important to the clinician is the anxiety generated by the family history: the patient with tiredness is concerned because his/her mother had SLE, or the patient with Raynaud's phenomenon is concerned because his/her mother had SSc. These fears/anxieties should not be underestimated.

### Social history

Smoking causes vascular injury, and therefore should be strongly discouraged in patients with connective tissue diseases who often already have a compromised vasculature. Details about occupation, housing, and social support are important to establish (as in other chronic diseases) whether or not a patient is able to work, and the level of home support, as these parameters are often major contributors to quality of life.

## Examination for signs of connective tissue disease

A full examination is required for the same reason as a full history: these are multisystem diseases and (in patients with established connective tissue disease or a vasculitis) drugs used in their treatment may cause a wide range of adverse effects.

### Systemic enquiry

#### General

Examine the temperature chart. As stated above, fever can be a manifestation of connective tissue disease. Many patients are anaemic and therefore pale. Lymphadenopathy is described in connective tissue disease but is uncommon, therefore other causes should also be considered (*Table 1.1*). In the patient with parotid gland enlargement, consider Sjögren's syndrome (**1.5**).

#### Skin and mucous membranes

The skin and mucous membranes should always be examined carefully because these can often give clues to an underlying connective tissue disease. Typical skin manifestations of the different connective tissue diseases are summarized in *Table 1.2*. While these have been listed by disease, it should be recognized that the skin and mucous membrane abnormalities overlap between diseases and so these are often false distinctions. For example, digital ischaemic ulcers can occur in SLE, SSc, and in the vasculitides.

- SLE. While the typical rash is facial ('butterfly') (**2.2A, B**) and photosensitive, more chronic lesions occur in discoid (**2.6, 2.7A**) and subacute cutaneous lupus erythematosus (**1.6**). Alopecia, which may be scarring especially in discoid lupus (**2.9**), and mouth ulcers are also common. Mouth ulcers are a common side-effect of immunosuppressant drugs and so this possibility should be considered where relevant.
- APS. This diagnosis should be considered in patients with livedo reticularis (**1.7**).
- SSc. This is associated with many different cutaneous manifestations:
- Skin thickening (scleroderma). Scleroderma proximal to the metacarpophalangeal joints is the major classification criterion for SSc and its development often leads to the diagnosis. Skin thickening usually begins in the fingers (sclerodactyly [**1.8**]), feet, and face and then may progress proximally especially in those with the diffuse cutaneous subtype. It must be remembered, however, that scleroderma occurs in conditions other than SSc and it is important to differentiate SSc from, for example, generalized morphoea (**1.9**) or eosinophilic fasciitis.

**1.5** Right-sided parotid gland enlargement in a patient with Sjögren's syndrome secondary to SSc.

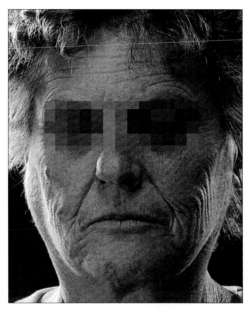

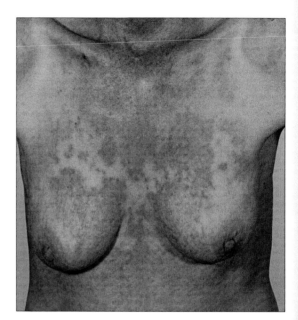

**1.6** Subacute cutaneous lupus erythematosus.

**1.7** Livedo reticularis. The rash is more obvious over the left knee than the right.

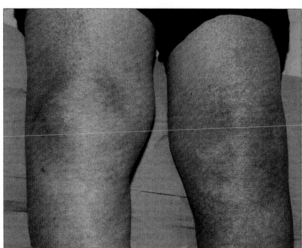

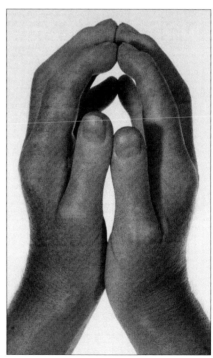

**1.9** Generalized morphoea, most marked over the thorax posteriorly where the skin is thickened, tight, and shiny. This is not SSc: the patient did not have Raynaud's phenomenon and the skin thickening did not commence distally.

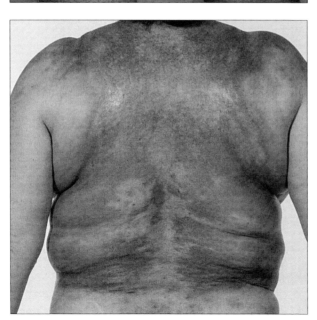

**1.8** Sclerodactyly. The skin is thickened, giving rise to flexion contractures of the fingers.

– Digital ulceration/ischaemia. An underlying connective tissue disease should always be suspected when a patient with good peripheral pulses presents with digital ulcers or ischaemia, because the pathology is likely to involve the digital arteries and/or the microvessels. Digital ulcers tend to occur at the fingertips in patients with limited cutaneous SSc (**1.10**) and over the proximal and distal interphalangeal joints in patients with diffuse cutaneous disease (**1.11**). Digital ulcers can become infected and severe digital ischaemia can progress to gangrene (**1.12**). Digital pitting (**1.13**) is one of the three minor classification criteria of SSc and reflects chronic digital ischaemia.

– Telangiectases (**1.14**). If accompanied by other characteristic symptoms and signs, for example, Raynaud's phenomenon, these should make one suspect SSc.

– Calcinosis. Subcutaneous calcinosis (**1.15**) should also always make one query an underlying diagnosis of SSc (**1.16**).

• Dermatomyositis. This diagnosis may be suspected from the typical rash, which commonly affects the face (sometimes with heliotrope discoloration and periorbital oedema, **5.5A, B**), neck and upper back, the extensor aspects of the hands (Gottron's papules, **5.6A, B**), elbows, and knees, and the periungal areas. Dermatomyositis is associated with marked abnormalities of the nailfold capillaries, which can sometimes be seen with the naked eye (**1.17A, B**).

• Vasculitis. Typical features pointing to an underlying vasculitis include splinter haemorrhages, nailfold infarcts, a purpuric rash (**1.18, 1.19A, B**) and vasculitic ulcers (**1.20A, B, 1.21**). If any of these are observed, then this should prompt a search for evidence of vasculitis elsewhere, for example renal vasculitis. As already mentioned, digital ischaemia and mouth ulcers (**1.2**) can also occur in the vasculitides. Because vasculitis can occur as part of other multisystem inflammatory diseases, for example in patients with rheumatoid arthritis and SLE, it is important always to be on the alert for signs of vasculitis because these might influence management (**1.21**).

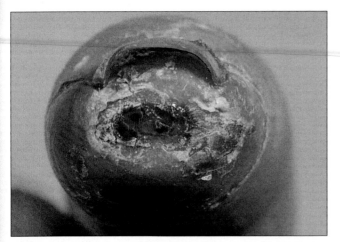

**1.10** Infected fingertip ulceration in a patient with limited cutaneous SSc.

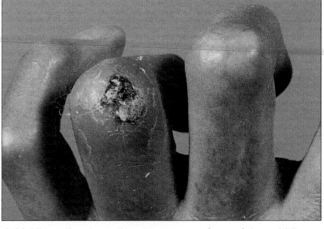

**1.11** Ulceration over the extensor surface of the middle finger proximal interphalangeal joint in a patient with diffuse cutaneous SSc. There is marked sclerodactyly with contractures.

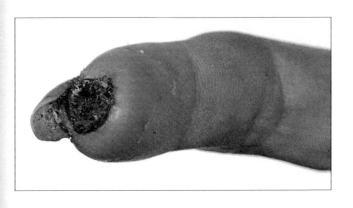

**1.12** Digital tip ulcer which has progressed to gangrene in a patient with SSc.

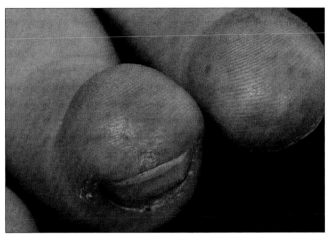

**1.13** Digital pitting (demonstrated in the finger on the left side of the image) in a patient with SSc.

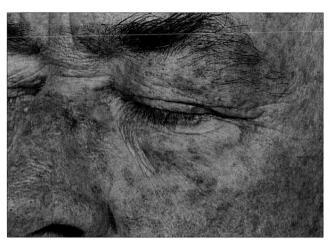

**1.14** Telangiectases in a patient with SSc.

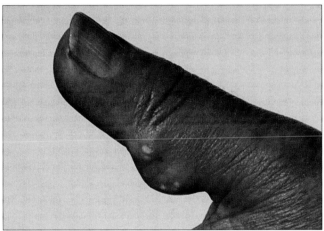

**1.15** Calcinosis of the thumb.

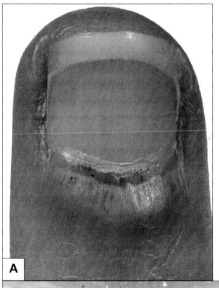

A

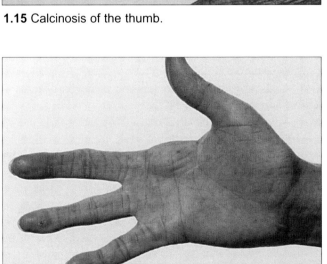

**1.16** Several clinical features of SSc: cyanosis of the middle and ring finger, digital pitting of the middle finger, a calcinotic nodule of the pulp of the ring finger, telangiectases, and amputation of the index finger (this was due to severe digital ischaemia).

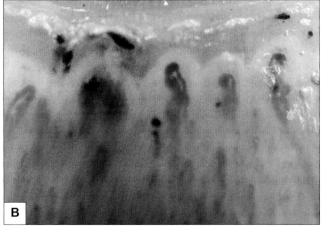

B

**1.17A**: Periungal erythema in a patient with probable early dermatomyositis. Dilated capillaries can be seen with the naked eye, as well as being well demonstrated with capillary microscopy (**B**).

**1.18** Purpuric rash of the lower limbs. Histology showed leucocytoclastic vasculitis.

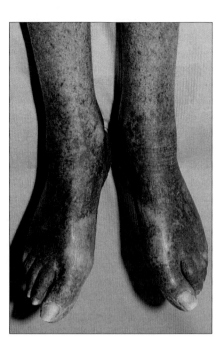

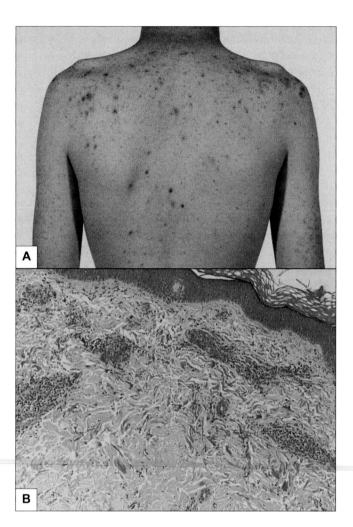

**1.19A**: Purpuric rash in a patient with Henoch–Schönlein purpura; **B**: histology of a skin biopsy from the patient shown in (**A**) shows superficial vessels surrounded and infiltrated by neutrophil polymorphs along with karyorrhectic debris. There is vascular damage with red blood cell extravasation. Magnification ×10. (Courtesy of Dr. L. Jamieson.)

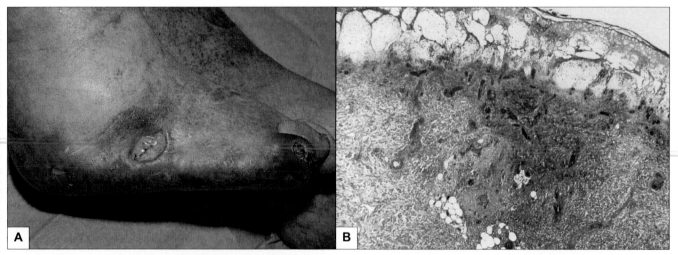

**1.20A**: Vasculitic ulcers, the most obvious one being over the lateral aspect of the midfoot. There is also a vasculitic rash of the left leg and ischaemic change of the right 5th toe; **B**: histology of one of the ulcers of the patient shown in (**A**) shows a dense leucocytoclastic neutrophilic infiltrate involving both large and small vessels leading to fibrinoid necrosis of the vessels as well as necrosis of the epidermis and striking papillary dermal oedema. Magnification ×4. (Courtesy of Dr. L. Jamieson.)

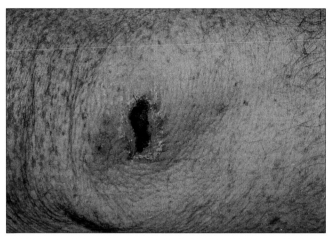

**1.21** Vasculitic ulcer in a patient with Wegener's granulomatosus. The sutures mark the site of the biopsy.

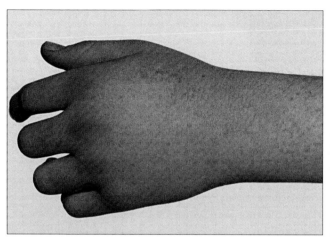

**1.22** Swelling of the dorsum of the hand and wrist due to arthritis in Henoch–Schönlein purpura. This is the same patient as in Figure **1.19**.

## Musculoskeletal

There are a large number of possible findings on musculoskeletal examination (*Table 1.3*), underscoring the need for a careful assessment in all patients in whom connective tissue disease is either confirmed or suspected. In inflammatory arthritis there is usually warmth, tenderness, and swelling (**1.22**). As with the skin, the characteristic musculoskeletal findings are considered under disease subheadings but again, this is a false distinction as there is considerable overlap in the possible manifestations between diseases.

- SLE. This is in the differential diagnosis in patients, especially young women, presenting with an inflammatory arthritis. There may be reversible deformities of the fingers.
- SSc. Contractures occur especially in patients with diffuse cutaneous disease (**1.8**). Patients with early diffuse disease may have friction rubs, for example at the knees and ankles.
- Inflammatory muscle disease. Pointers to the diagnosis are proximal muscle weakness and tenderness.

As a final point, fibromyalgia can occur in patients with connective tissue disease so if a patient has multiple tender points then this diagnosis should be considered.

## Cardiorespiratory

Key points to look for in patients with suspected or proven connective tissue disease are shown in *Table 1.4* and include:

- Raised blood pressure. This may reflect renal involvement or concomitant 'essential' hypertension. Either way, it is imperative that the blood pressure be well controlled. Hypertension in a patient with SSc may may occur in 'scleroderma renal crisis', which is a medical emergency; therefore, the blood pressure must be checked in any patient with SSc who develops new symptoms such as headache or new breathlessness.
- A loud pulmonary component to the second heart sound, suggesting pulmonary hypertension.
- Basal crackles, suggesting pulmonary fibrosis.

## Gastrointestinal

Key points to look for include signs of weight loss, abdominal tenderness (which can occur in SLE-related serositis or in patients with mesenteric ischaemia), and abdominal distension (which can occur in patients with SSc and episodes of pseudo-obstruction secondary to small bowel involvement).

## Nervous system

Connective tissue diseases can give rise to a wide spectrum of neurological signs reflecting how peripheral, central, and autonomic nervous systems can all be involved (*Table 1.6*). Points to highlight are as follows:

- If a patient has signs of mononeuritis multiplex, consider whether he/she might have vasculitis.
- Peripheral neuropathy (which may be asymptomatic) may be a feature of several of the connective tissue diseases.

- Trigeminal neuropathy, clinical features of which include impaired sensation in the distribution of one or more branches of the trigeminal nerve, may be the presenting feature of connective tissue disease.
- Meningitis should always be suspected in the unwell patient with SLE, for example with drowsiness and pyrexia. The immediate concern is bacterial meningitis, although aseptic meningitis can also occur in SLE.

### Eyes

Abnormalities include redness in the patient with conjunctivitis or uveitis (for example in Behçet's disease), abnormalities of the sclera in vasculitis, and proptosis in Wegener's granulomatosis. The fundi should be examined if there is any possibility of retinal vasculitis, for example in the patient with SLE, in whom cotton wool exudates may be found.

## Investigations in a patient with suspected connective tissue disease

As a generalization, investigations are indicated to:
- *Inform diagnosis.* Some investigations are highly specific for different connective tissue diseases. For example, a diffuse cANCA staining is very suggestive of Wegener's granulomatosis. The finding of histological vasculitis will confirm a suspected diagnosis and may give confidence to the clinician that immunosuppressant therapy is justified.
- *Monitor disease activity.* Monitoring of the acute phase response (ESR and/or C-reactive protein [CRP]) is standard practice in assessing disease activity/treatment response in most of the connective tissue diseases. In certain connective tissue diseases, monitoring levels of certain specific autoantibodies can also be useful (for example cANCA in Wegener's granulomatosis or anti-double-stranded DNA [dsDNA] antibodies in patients with SLE).

Because connective tissue diseases, including the vasculitides, are often complex and multisystem, a large number of investigations may be required in any one individual, firstly at the time of diagnosis, and secondly in the monitoring of disease activity/severity and in the documentation of the degree of involvement (if any) of the different internal organs. Therefore, it is not possible to give a comprehensive list of all the investigations which might be required, nor of all the possible abnormalities. This section will give a summary of some of the tests which are most frequently requested/helpful. Most patients with a proven or suspected diagnosis of connective tissue disease will, on presentation, require the following investigative 'work-up':
- A full blood count.
- A biochemical profile.
- Assay of an acute phase reactant, usually the ESR or CRP.
- Dipstick testing of urine, and microscopy of urine.
- Immunology testing, including ANA.
- A chest X-ray.
- Other tests as clinically indicated.

The broad principles will be discussed here.

### Tests
#### Haematology

Patients with active connective tissue disease typically have a normochromic normocytic anaemia, a slightly raised platelet count, and a raised ESR. However, this is not true of patients with 'primary' APS (i.e. not associated with a connective tissue disease such as SLE) and SSc, which are not usually associated with a major inflammatory component. A high ESR in the patient with SSc should make one query whether there is an overlap with another connective tissue disease, or whether there is an additional pathology such as infection or malignancy.

Active SLE may be associated with a fall in the haemoglobin, white cell count, and/or platelet count. A proportion of patients with SLE develop autoimmune haemolytic anaemia. Thrombocytopenia occurs in APS. Eosinophilia occurs in Churg–Strauss syndrome.

It is essential to monitor the full blood count in patients on immunosuppressive therapy. A fall in any of the components of the blood count should alert the clinician to the possibility of drug toxicity. As already discussed above, a common clinical dilemma is the patient with SLE and pancytopenia. Bone marrow examination may be helpful.

#### Blood biochemistry
- Blood biochemical profile. This should always be checked. Many patients with connective tissue disease have renal or (less frequently) hepatic involvement which may be asymptomatic.
- CRP. This is typically raised in active inflammation, although not usually elevated in SLE unless there is serositis. Therefore, a raised CRP in the patient with SLE should always prompt the clinician to look for underlying infection.
- Muscle enzymes. These should always be checked if an inflammatory muscle disease is suspected. Creatine phosphokinase is most commonly used in diagnosis and

**Table 1.7 Autoantibody associations with connective tissue diseases[1]**

*SLE*
- Anti-dsDNA antibodies. Highly specific for SLE. Titre can be a useful measure of disease activity. However, not sensitive: many patients with SLE do not demonstrate anti-dsDNA antibodies
- Anti-Sm antibodies. Specific, not sensitive
- Anti-Ro and anti-La antibodies (associated with Sjögren's sydrome as below). Not sensitive. Both these autoantibodies are associated with the neonatal lupus syndrome and so women of childbearing age with either of these antibodies need to be advised accordingly and ideally should have prepregnancy counselling

*Sjögren's syndrome*
- Anti-Ro and anti-La antibodies

*APS*
- Anti-cardiolipin antibodies. Low levels of anti-cardiolipin antibodies occur in a number of other clinical situations (e.g. infection) and so this finding is not specific

*SSc*
- Anti-centromere antibodies (in limited cutaneous disease). Specific, but not sensitive
- Anti-topoisomerase (anti-Scl-70) antibodies (in diffuse cutaneous disease, with an association with pulmonary fibrosis). Specific, but not sensitive

- Anti-RNA polymerase I and III antibodies (in diffuse cutaneous disease, with an association with renal involvement). Specific, but not sensitive

*Inflammatory muscle disease*
- Anti-Jo-1 antibodies (associated with lung fibrosis). Specific, not sensitive[2]
- Anti-PM-Scl antibodies (associated with SSc overlap)

*Vasculitis*
- cANCA (associated with Wegener's granulomatosis). Antibody is usually to proteinase 3. Specific, not sensitive
- Perinuclear ANCA (pANCA). Less specific than cANCA for vasculitis. Antibody is usually to myeloperoxidase

*Overlap syndromes*
- U1 RNP antibodies. This antibody must, by definition, be present for the diagnosis of mixed connective tissue disease

[1]This list is not comprehensive but includes the autoantibodies currently most useful to the practising clinician. For example, a large number of different autoantibodies are now recognized to be associated with inflammatory muscle disease
[2]A number of other anti-synthetase antibodies are now recognized. Anti-Jo-1 is the one most commonly found

monitoring: blood levels may be very high on presentation with polymyositis. Circulating levels of aldolase, transaminases, and lactate dehydrogenase may all be high in patients with muscle inflammation.
- Globulins. Hypergammaglobulinaemia (polyclonal) may be seen especially in patients with Sjögren's syndrome.

### Urine

All patients with a suspected or proven diagnosis of connective tissue disease should have dipstick testing of urine. So often this simple test is omitted or delayed (Scenario 1) yet an abnormal dipstick may be the first clue to renal involvement. Glomerulonephritis can occur in SLE or the vasculitides. Dipstick testing may then show protein and/or blood, and microscopy of urine an active sediment with white and red blood cells and casts. If renal

involvement is suspected, then a urine sample should be sent for estimation of protein/creatine ratio and for creatinine clearance.

### Immunology

The connective tissue diseases are associated with circulating autoantibodies and as already stated these can be useful in diagnosis. Also, in individual connective tissue diseases, particular autoantibodies are associated with certain phenotypes. For example, in patients with SSc, anti-centromere antibody is highly specific (but not sensitive) for the limited cutaneous disease subtype whereas anti-topoisomerase (anti-Scl-70) is specific (but not sensitive) for the diffuse cutaneous subtype. Some of the autoantibody associations with the different connective tissue diseases are listed in *Table 1.7*.

If a patient presents with what could be a connective tissue disease (e.g. fever, rash, splinter haemorrhages, anaemia, and a raised ESR), one or more of the following immunological tests are indicated, depending on the clinical context:

- ANA. This is a nonspecific test but useful in screening. Over 95% of patients with SLE are ANA positive. The higher the titre, the more likely the patient is to have an autoimmune disease: an ANA titre of 1/1,600 is much more likely to be clinically relevant than a titre of 1/100.
- Antibodies to dsDNA. These should be assayed if the ANA is positive and the patient is suspected of having SLE. The level of anti-dsDNA antibodies can be a useful measure of disease activity.
- Antibodies to specific antigens. These are more disease-specific than the ANA. Some useful disease/auto-antibody associations are listed in *Table 1.7*. As a generalization, most of the disease-specific auto-antibodies are not sensitive, i.e. many patients with the disease do not have the autoantibody.
- Cryoglobulins. These are proteins that precipitate when cold, and can occur in connective tissue disease and vasculitis, infections (particularly hepatitis C), or malignancy. Cryoglobulins may be monoclonal (in which case myeloma or another haematological malignancy should be suspected), polyclonal, or 'mixed'.
- Testing for APS. Testing for both lupus anticoagulant (a functional assay which measures the ability of a patient's serum to prolong *in vitro* measures of clotting) and anti-cardiolipin antibodies should be requested if a patient is suspected of having an APS. This is because one test may be negative but the other positive.

### Other investigations
These will be indicated according to the clinical picture. However, some general points can be made.

### Investigation of suspected muscle inflammation
The muscle enzymes should be checked as above. Other tests are: electromyography (EMG), muscle biopsy, and magnetic resonance (MR) scanning (**1.23A, B**). An important clinical point is that a normal muscle biopsy does not exclude the diagnosis of inflammatory muscle disease because the myositic process is patchy and may be missed on biopsy.

### Investigation of suspected vasculitis
The 'gold standard' investigation is biopsy, as appearances may be diagnostic. Sometimes the histological appearances will point to a specific type of vasculitis. For example, a necrotizing granulomatous vasculitis affecting small and medium vessels would be highly suggestive of Wegener's granulomatosis. The site of the biopsy will depend upon the clinical scenario. For example, renal biopsy was indicated in Scenario 1 because of the renal impairment and the haematuria and proteinuria. Other common biopsy sites are skin, sural nerve, temporal artery (if temporal arteritis is suspected), and muscle. Angiography may also play a key role in the diagnosis and assessment of vasculitis. For example, if a diagnosis of vasculitis is suspected in a patient with abdominal pain, then the finding of aneurysms and/or vascular occlusions on mesenteric angiography may point to a diagnosis of polyarteritis nodosa. Newer techniques, including MR and computed tomographic (CT) angiography, which are less invasive than conventional (X-ray) angiography, are now used in the monitoring of large-vessel vasculitis such as Takayasu's arteritis.

### Investigation of the patient with Raynaud's phenomenon
In the patient with primary (idiopathic) Raynaud's phenomenon, there should be no symptoms or signs suggestive of an underlying connective tissue disease. In addition, the ANA should be negative or present in low titre only (<1/100), the ESR should be normal, and the nailfold capillaries should be normal. Nailfold capillaroscopy is believed to be the investigation best predictive of underlying connective tissue disease, abnormal capillaries (**1.24A, B**) conferring a relative risk of an underlying SSc (or 'scleroderma')-spectrum disorder in the order of 13.

### Other investigations to identify presence and degree of internal organ involvement
It is not possible to provide a comprehensive list, as the multisystem and heterogeneous nature of the connective tissue diseases means that almost any investigation might be required. Some challenging and relatively common clinical scenarios are as follows:

- Investigation of breathlessness in a patient with SLE or other connective tissue disease. The differential diagnosis is extensive, but investigations will include a chest X-ray (**1.25, 1.26**), pulmonary function tests with transfer factor, an electrocardiogram (ECG) (**1.27**), an echocardiogram (to include estimation of the pulmonary artery pressure), and most likely a high-resolution CT scan of the thorax.
- Investigation of weight loss in a patient with SSc or other connective tissue disease. Weight loss is often multifactorial and has several possible causes. Investigation in the patient with SSc should include checking for bacterial overgrowth with hydrogen and [$^{14}$C] labelled breath test.

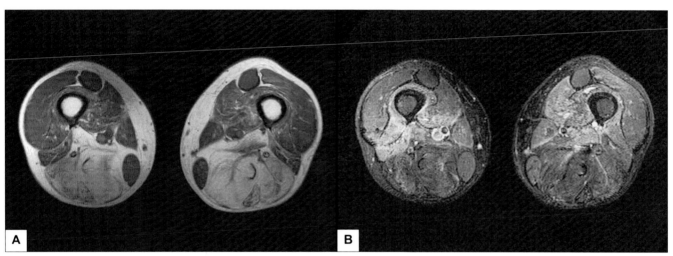

**1.23** MR images showing myositis. **A**: T1-weighted image shows the replacement of the posterior muscle groups with fat, fat atrophy; **B**: STIR image shows the muscle as patchy high signal, indicating an increase in the muscle water content (oedema). (Courtesy of Dr. C. Hutchinson.)

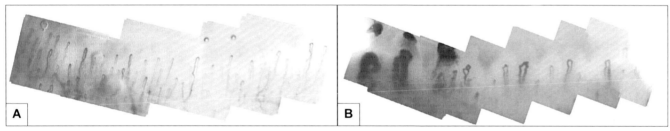

**1.24** Normal (**A**) and abnormal (**B**) capillaroscopy in a patient with SSc, showing dilated loops and (left side of image) giant capillaries and areas of haemorrhage.

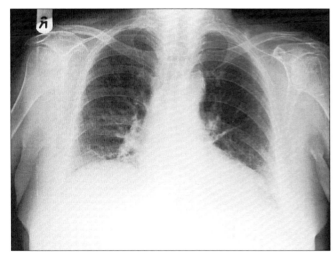

**1.25** Chest X-ray showing basal shadowing (pulmonary fibrosis) in a patient with SLE.

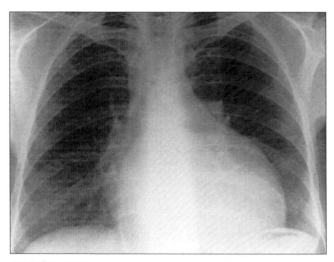

**1.26** Chest X-ray showing pericardial effusion in a patient with SSc. The patient was breathless and the pericardial effusion was drained.

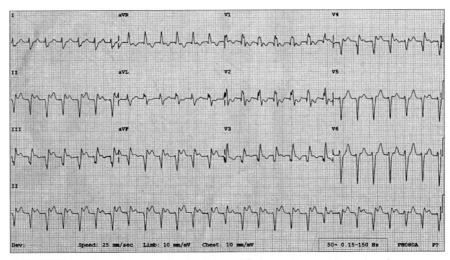

**1.27** ECG in a breathless patient with an SSc/myositis overlap, showing supraventricular tachycardia.

- Investigation of lethargy in a patient with connective tissue disease. A common clinical dilemma is to decide how far to pursue the symptom of fatigue, which is one of the main symptoms of connective tissue disease and yet which can have other causes. It is not possible to generalize, but it is important to remember that patients with autoimmune connective tissue disease have an increased prevalence of thyroid disease over the general population, and are often anaemic via a variety of possible mechanisms. The key is a careful clinical assessment.

## Conclusions

Assessment of patients with connective tissue diseases including the vasculitides is complex. Even once a diagnosis is made, the disease course is often unpredictable and for that reason most patients will require long-term follow-up, often involving more than one specialist. A detailed history and examination, backed up by relevant investigations, are key factors in defining the problem at any one point in time so that an appropriate management strategy may be followed. Any new symptom or sign must be pursued. Even if not directly attributable to the underlying connective tissue disease, any comorbidity and its treatment may impact on the patient, underscoring the need for a holistic approach to investigation and management.

## Further reading

Cutolo M, Grassi W, Matucci Cerinic M (2003). Raynaud's phenomenon and the role of capillaroscopy. *Arthr Rheum* **11**:3023–30.

Kumar TS, Aggarwal A (2010). Approach to a patient with connective tissue disease. *Indian J Paediatr* 77:1157–64.

LeRoy EC, Medsger TA (1992). Raynaud's phenomenon: a proposal for classification. *Clin Exp Rheumatol* **10**:485–8.

McLuskey P, Powell RJ (2004). The eye in systemic inflammatory diseases. *Lancet* **364**:2125–33.

Solomon DH, Kavanaugh AJ, Schur PH (2002). Evidence-based guidelines for the use of immunological tests: antinuclear antibody testing. *Arthr Rheum (Arthr Care Res)* 47(4):434–44.

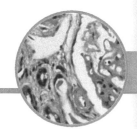

# Systemic lupus erythematosus

*Caroline Gordon, Julia U Holle, and Wolfgang L Gross*

## Definition and pathology

Systemic lupus erythematosus (SLE) is a complex, multisystemic autoimmune disease associated with the presence of autoantibodies and characterized by remissions and relapses that can present with a variety of clinical manifestations. It is part of a spectrum of autoimmune diseases that also includes Sjögren's syndrome, anti-phospholipid syndrome (APS), dermatomyositis/poly-myositis, and overlap syndromes which will be discussed in subsequent chapters.

SLE is characterized by multiple immune abnormalities involving B and T cells and dendritic dysfunction resulting in the development of autoantibodies and autoreactive T cells. The presence of certain autoantibodies in the serum forms the basis of tests for diagnosis and monitoring of the disease as described below. Defective clearance of apoptotic cells (particularly after ultraviolet [UV] light exposure or infection) and of immune complexes contributes to pathogenesis. Complement activation by immune complexes is an important mediator of tissue damage and complement consumption can be used to assess disease activity (see below). The cytokine interferon-alpha (IFN-$\alpha$) appears to play a role in activating genes involved in the development of the disease and the cytokines IFN-$\alpha$, interleukin (IL)-6 and IL-10 are increased in the serum of patients with active disease. Anti-phospholipid antibodies are a specific family of autoantibodies directed against anionic phospholipids in cell membranes that are prothrombotic. These antibodies may occur in SLE and in primary APS, which is discussed in Chapter 4.

## Epidemiology

### Associations with age and gender

SLE is a multifactorial disease associated with genetic and environmental factors that are still not well understood and vary between affected individuals. Lupus is a disease that affects predominantly women in the reproductive age group. However, the disease can start in childhood, though it is uncommon before puberty, and in males of any age. It has also been increasingly recognized to occur in postmeno-pausal women, particularly in Caucasians. Manifestations of lupus present at diagnosis vary with age (*Table 2.1*).

### Distribution worldwide and role of ethnicity

SLE is a disease that occurs worldwide but is more common and often more severe in certain racial groups,

| Table 2.1 Differences in lupus manifestations at time of diagnosis between children and adults |||
|---|---|---|
| **Item** | **% Children** | **% Adults** |
| Fever | 41–76 | 21 |
| Lymphadenopathy | 6–72 | 0.5 |
| Renal | 20–67 | 9–33 |
| Gastrointestinal | 25 | NR |
| Neurological | 0–25 | 6–10 |
| Haematological | 38–58 | 16 |
| Sicca symptoms | 0 | 17 |

**Table 2.2 Prevalence of lupus by country in various studies undertaken since 1990 worldwide**

| Continent | Country | Ethnic groups* | Prevalence per 100,000 |
|---|---|---|---|
| America | US | C | 122 |
| | US | AA, C | 124 |
| | US | H | 103 |
| | US | AA, C | 241 |
| Europe | Sweden | C | 68 |
| | UK | AC, C, A | 28 |
| | Finland | C | 28 |
| | UK | AC, C | 25 |
| | Ireland | C | 25 |
| | Denmark | C | 22 |
| | Norway | C | 45 |
| Oceania | Australia | AAu, C | 45 |
| Asia | Saudi Arabia | A (Arabic) | 19 |

*A: Asian; AA: African-American; AAu: Aboriginal Australian; AC: African-Caribbean; C: Caucasian; H: Hispanic

such as those of African descent in North America or the Caribbean and those from around the Pacific rim including those from the Far East, the Indian subcontinent, and those of Polynesian origin. The prevalence and incidence of lupus vary with the ethnic composition of the population studied, the geographical location, and at different ages, and are summarized in *Tables 2.2–2.5.*

**Table 2.3 Prevalence and incidence of lupus in Birmingham, UK, in different ethnic groups**

| Group | Prevalence (per 100,000) | Incidence (per 100,000) |
|---|---|---|
| Adults | 27.7 | 3.8 |
| Adult women | 49.6 | 6.8 |
| Caucasian women | 36.3 | 2.5–3.4 |
| African-Caribbean women | 197.2 | 11.9–31.9 |
| South Asian women | 96.5 | 4.1–15.2 |

**Table 2.4 Prevalence and incidence of lupus in USA in different ethnic groups**

| Group | Prevalence (per 100,000) | Incidence (per 100,000) |
|---|---|---|
| Adults | 4.8–78.5 | 0.7–7.2 |
| Adult women | 7.7–131.5 | 1.1–11.4 |
| Caucasians | 4.8–9.9 | 0.7–2.2 |
| African-Americans | 9.3–29.6 | 1.7–7.2 |
| Puerto Ricans | 18.0 | 2.3 |

**Table 2.5 Incidence of SLE in females in ethnic groups and with age**

| Ethnic group | Diagnosis at age <10 yrs (per 100,000) | Diagnosis at age ≥10 yrs (per 100,000) |
|---|---|---|
| Hispanics | 4.6 | 13.0 |
| African-Americans | 3.7 | 19.9 |
| Asians (Chinese) | 6.2 | 31.1 |

## Environmental factors

SLE is associated with flares (relapses) and remissions. Flares are often triggered by exposure to UV light, infection, hormonal changes, and stress. There is increasing evidence that the disease is caused by environmental influences acting on a complex genetic background. Potential predisposing factors in the environment are summarized in *Table 2.6*. In the past, not only was disease onset related to the hormonal changes of puberty or pregnancy in many cases but administration of exogenous oestrogens appeared to induce the disease or cause flares (oestrogen-containing contraceptives or hormone replacement therapy). Recent studies have shown, however, that women with well-controlled mild or moderate disease and with no prothrombotic tendency can be given such hormonal therapies without risk of severe flares.

## Genetic predisposition

The genetic predisposition to lupus involves between 20 and 40 genes. Even in identical twins the risk of both twins developing lupus is about 25%, emphasizing the role of the environment in addition to the genetic background. The risk of developing lupus in first-degree relatives of an affected individual is about 5% (1 in 20). The best-known genetic risk factors are in the major histocompatibility complex, particularly the haplotype HLA-A1, B8, C4 null, DR3. The genes most associated with SLE are shown in *Table 2.7*. Recent studies have suggested that a number of genes associated with immune responses are involved in the predisposition to lupus, including immunoglobulin receptors (FCGR2A and FCGR3B), complement (C1q), and cytokines such as tumour necrosis factor (TNF), interferon (IFN) regulatory factor 5 (IRF5), integrins (ITGAM), B lymphoid tyrosine kinase (BLK), important in B cell signalling and induction of autoantibodies, transcription activator STAT4, and protein tyrosine phosphatase nonreceptor 22 (PTPN22), involved in down-regulation of T cell activation.

### Table 2.6 Environmental influences on the development of SLE

| Environmental agent | Examples |
| --- | --- |
| Ultraviolet light | UV-A and UV-B |
| Infections | Viruses such as CMV, EBV, parvovirus B19, retroviruses* |
| Hormones | Oestrogens |
| | Prolactin |
| Drugs | Minocycline and other tetracyclines |
| | Sulphonamides including sulphasalazine |
| | Isoniazid |
| | Penicillamine |
| | Hydralazine, procainamide |
| | Phenytoin, carbamazepine |
| | Chlorpromazine |
| Heavy metals | Mercury |
| | Cadmium* |
| Chemicals | Crystalline silica |
| | Pesticides* |
| | Solvents* |
| Dietary factors | L-canavanine in alfalfa* |

*Not confirmed

### Table 2.7 Genes most associated with development of SLE and the level of evidence as measured by risk ratio

| Candidate genes | Risk ratio |
| --- | --- |
| MHC | 2.36 |
| ITGAM | 1.62 |
| IRF5 | 1.54 |
| BLK | 1.39 |
| STAT4 | 1.53 |
| PTPN22 | 1.53 |
| FCGR2A | 1.35 |

BLK: a B lymphoid–specific tyrosine kinase of the Src family; FCGR2A: immunoglobulin Fc gamma receptor 2A; IRF5: interferon regulatory factor 5; ITGAM: intergrin-alpha M (also known as CD11b); MHC: major histocompatibility complex; PTPN22: protein tyrosine phosphatase nonreceptor 22; STAT4: signal transduction and activator of transcription 4

### Outcome and causes of death

Over the last 50 years there has been an improvement in survival in SLE patients (**2.1**). From about 50% survival at 5 years after diagnosis in the 1950s, survival figures of about 97% at 5 years and 91% at 10 years have been reported in Europe in the last 10 years. Prognosis for patients with renal involvement, African descent, and poor socioeconomic background has been less good than for patients without these factors, and 10-year survival rates of about 80% have been found in North American populations and of about 50% in India and Taiwan. The main causes of death are increasingly infection and cardiovascular disease (especially premature atherosclerosis secondary to lupus), though in countries where access to good health care may be limited by availability or cost there are still considerable numbers of deaths due to lupus activity and renal failure. The commonest causes of death in SLE patients and frequency compared to that expected for age and gender, expressed as standardized mortality ratio, in the largest worldwide study by the Systemic Lupus International Collaborating Clinics is shown in *Table 2.8*. Non-Hodgkin's lymphoma (NHL) and lung cancer in smokers have been found to occur more frequently than expected in lupus patients. To date there is no definite evidence that immunosuppression increases the risk of malignancy in lupus patients.

## Presentation of systemic lupus

This multisystem disease may present as a slowly progressive condition with an increasing number of systems involved, initially relatively mildly, over several years or as a rapidly progressive condition with several systems involved more severely over a few weeks or months. There is a variety of clinical and laboratory manifestations that may accumulate over time, and the frequency of each is summarized in *Table 2.9*. These are discussed further in the sections below. Some of the most distinguishing features of lupus are included in the American College of Rheumatology (formerly the American Rheumatological Association) classification criteria for SLE (see *Table 2.10*). To be classified as having lupus requires the patient to have had four or more criteria over time. These criteria are sometimes considered to be diagnostic criteria for lupus but they were designed as classification criteria to be used to determine which patients can be entered into lupus clinical trials and outcome studies. Diagnosis of lupus is discussed further below.

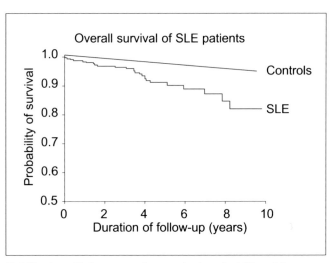

**2.1** Kaplan–Meier curve for survival probability of the Birmingham SLE cohort compared to age and sex adjusted local population estimates in 2001.

**Table 2.8 Commonest causes of death in SLE patients and frequency compared to that expected for age and gender, expressed as standardized mortality ratio**

| Cause of death | Standardized mortality ratio | |
|---|---|---|
| | SMR | (95% confidence intervals) |
| All | 2.4 | 2.3–2.5 |
| Circulatory | 1.7 | 1.5–1.9 |
|   Heart | 1.7 | 1.4–2.0 |
|   Stroke | 1.1 | 0.7–1.7 |
| Malignancy | 0.8 | 0.6–1.0 |
|   NHL | 2.8 | 1.2–5.6 |
|   Lung cancer | 2.3 | 1.6–3.0 |
| Infections | 5.0 | 3.7–6.7 |
| Pneumonia | 2.6 | 1.6–4.1 |
| Other respiratory causes | 1.3 | 0.8–1.6 |
| Renal disease | 7.9 | 5.5–11.0 |

NHL: non-Hodgkin's lymphoma

### Table 2.9 Cumulative percentage incidence of typical features of systemic lupus erythematosus

| Feature | % SLE patients | Feature | % SLE patients |
|---|---|---|---|
| Alopecia | 52–80 | Immunological | 60–77 |
| ANA | 96–99 | Malar rash | 37–90 |
| Arthritis | 72–94 | Neuropsychiatric | 6–63 |
| Cardiac | 10–29 | Oral/nasal ulcers | 30–61 |
| Discoid rash | 10–14 | Photosensitivity | 10–62 |
| Fever | 74–91 | Pleuropulmonary | 9–54 |
| Haematological | 61–90 | | |

### Table 2.10 Revised criteria of the American College of Rheumatology for the classification of SLE

**Malar rash**

Fixed erythema, flat or raised, over the malar eminences tending to spare the nasolabial folds

**Discoid rash**

Erythematosus raised patches with adherent keratotic scaling and follicular plugging; atrophic scarring may occur in older lesions

**Photosensitivity**

Skin rash as a result of unusual reaction to sunlight, by patient history or physician observation

**Oral ulcers**

Oral or nasopharyngeal ulceration, usually painless, observed by a physician

**Arthritis**

Nonerosive arthritis involving two or more peripheral joints, characterized by tenderness, swelling, or effusion

**Serositis**

• Pleuritis – convincing history of pleuritic pain or rub heard by a physician or evidence of pleural effusion OR
• Pericarditis – documented by ECG or rub or evidence of pericardial effusion

**Renal disorder**

• Persistent proteinuria greater than 0.5 g/day or greater than 3+ if quantification not performed OR
• Cellular casts – may be red cell, haemoglobin, granular, tubular or mixed

**Neurologic disorder**

• Seizures – in the absence of offending drugs or known metabolic derangements, e.g. uraemia, ketoacidosis, OR electrolyte imbalance OR
• Psychosis – in the absence of offending drugs or known metabolic derangements, e.g. uraemia, ketoacidosis, OR electrolyte imbalance

**Hematologic disorder**

• Haemolytic anaemia – with reticulocytosis OR
• Leukopenia – less than 4000/mm$^3$ OR
• Lymphopenia – less than 1500/mm$^3$ OR
• Thrombocytopenia – less than 1500/mm$^3$

**Immunologic disorder**

• Anti-DNA: antibody to native DNA in abnormal titre OR
• Anti-Sm: presence of antibody to Sm nuclear antigen OR
• Positive finding of anti-phospholipid antibodies based on: (1) an abnormal serum level of IgG or IgM anti-cardiolipin antibodies; (2) a positive test for lupus anticoagulant using a standard method; or (3) a false positive test for at least 6 months and confirmed by *Treponema pallidum* immobilization or fluorescent antibody absorption test

**Positive ANA**

An abnormal titre of ANA by immunofluorescence or an equivalent assay at any point in time in the absence of drugs

The incidence of each feature shown in *Tables 2.1* and *2.9* varies in the literature because the composition of the lupus cohorts reported in the literature vary in terms of the patients' ethnicity, age at enrolment to the cohort, duration of follow-up, access to cohort (insurance issues in some cases), and nature of the cohort (primary, secondary, or tertiary care or mixed). Some of the differences in lupus manifestations between Caucasians and non-Caucasians (African-American or South Asian from India/Pakistan) seen in Birmingham, UK, are shown in *Table 2.11*. Renal disease and serositis are common in non-Caucasians whereas photosensitivity is most common in Caucasians.

When assessing lupus patients it is important to distinguish reversible inflammatory disease from thrombotic complications of APS and from chronic damage due to the accumulated effects of the disease and its therapy, for example, lung fibrosis, myocardial infarction, or cataracts. The possibility of infection and other comorbid conditions should always be considered, not least of all because infection is a common trigger for lupus. Other factors that may induce flares of active disease include UV exposure, hormonal changes (oestrogens), and stress (for example major life events).

## Systemic enquiry
### General

The most common complaint and one of the hardest to treat is fatigue. It may be associated with depression or fibromyalgia, hypothyroidism (often autoimmune in nature), anaemia, pulmonary or cardiovascular problems. Other constitutional symptoms of active lupus that may occur include fever, anorexia, lymphadenopathy, and weight loss. These cannot be attributed to lupus until infection and malignancy have been excluded.

### Mucocutaneous manifestations

The best-known features of lupus are photosensitive rashes and the butterfly or malar rash on the face (**2.2A, B**). Other common mucocutaneous features are painful or painless mouth ulcers (**2.3**), diffuse alopecia (spontaneous hair loss) which may be localized (**2.4A, B**) or more diffuse (**2.4C**). Other typical rashes include subacute cutaneous lupus erythematosus (**2.5**) and discoid lupus rash (**2.6A, B**). Discoid lesions often cause scarring and may heal with hypopigmentation or hyperpigmentation (**2.7A** and **2.7B**, respectively). Scarring alopecia may occur in association with discoid rash in the scalp (**2.8A, B, 2.9**). Nasal or vaginal ulcers may also occur but are less common than oral ulcers.

**Table 2.11 Differences in the cumulative incidence of the American College of Rheumatology classification criteria for SLE between Caucasian and non-Caucasian patients in Birmingham, UK**

|  | Number of patients (%) | | | |
|---|---|---|---|---|
|  | All (n=333) | Caucasians (n=190) | Non-Caucasians (n=143) | P-value |
| Malar rash | 142 (42.6%) | 80 (42.1%) | 62 (43.4%) | 0.91 |
| Discoid rash | 36 (10.8%) | 18 (9.5%) | 18 (12.6%) | 0.47 |
| Photosensitivity | 166 (49.8%) | 111 (58.4%) | 55 (38.5%) | <0.001* |
| Oral ulcers | 192 (57.7%) | 107 (56.3%) | 85 (59.4%) | 0.65 |
| Arthritis | 314 (94.3%) | 182 (95.8%) | 132 (92.3%) | 0.26 |
| Serositis | 114 (34.2%) | 53 (27.9%) | 61 (42.7%) | 0.01* |
| Renal | 74 (22.2%) | 33 (17.4%) | 41 (28.7%) | 0.02* |
| Neurological | 33 (9.9%) | 14 (7.4%) | 19 (13.3%) | 0.11 |
| Haematological | 252 (75.7%) | 135 (71.1%) | 117 (81.8%) | 0.03* |
| Immunological | 218 (65.5%) | 119 (62.6%) | 99 (69.2%) | 0.26 |
| ANA positivity | 321 (96.4%) | 182 (95.8%) | 135 (94.4%) | 0.55 |

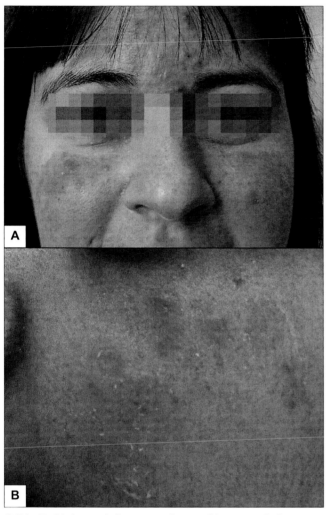

**2.2A, B**: Malar rash in two patients with systemic lupus erythematosus (front and side views).

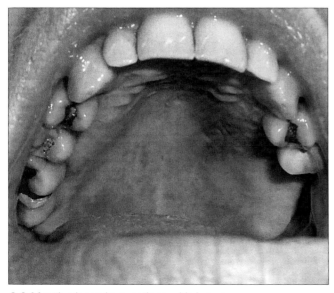

**2.3** Mouth ulcers in a patient with lupus.

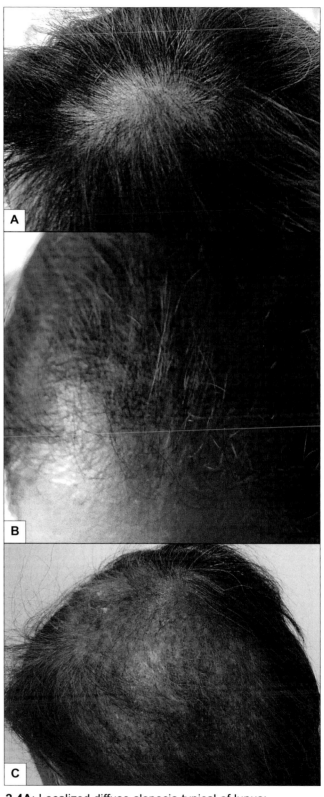

**2.4A**: Localized diffuse alopecia typical of lupus;
**B**: frontal hair loss and 'frizz' typical of lupus;
**C**: severe diffuse alopecia due to lupus with signs of new hair growth.

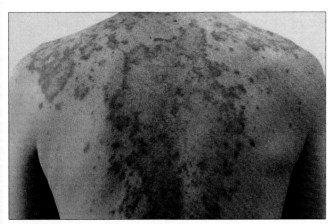

**2.5** The rash of subacute cutaneous lupus erythematosus.

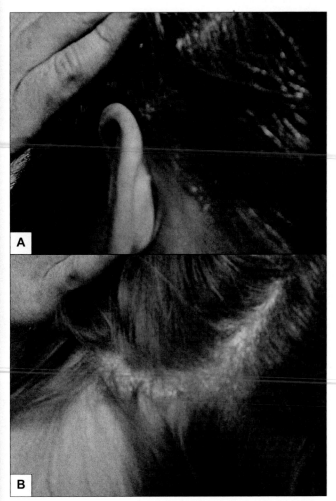

**2.6** Recent onset discoid rash in the scalp (**A**) and at the hair line (**B**).

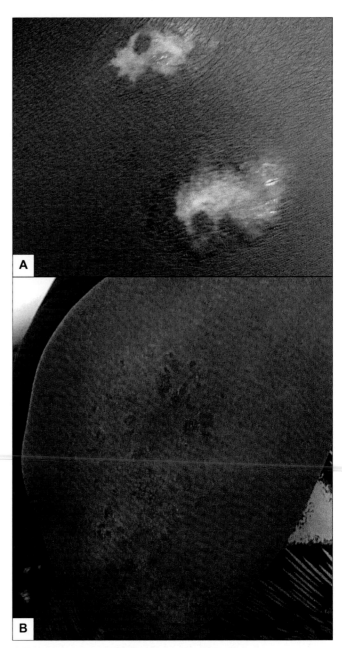

**2.7A**: Hypopigmentation from scarring discoid rash; **B**: hyperpigmentation from lupus rash.

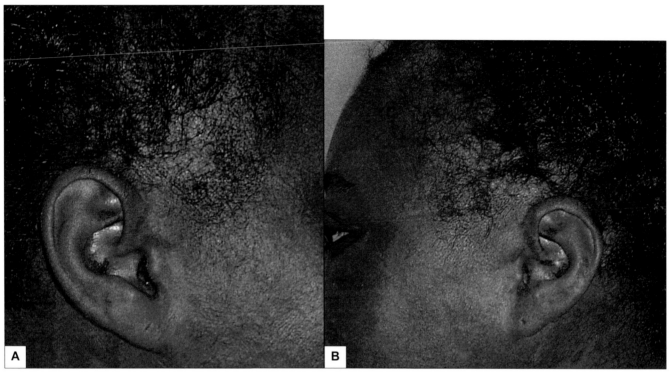

**2.8A, B**: Hyperpimentation and hair loss associated with discoid lupus rash in an Afro-Caribbean woman.

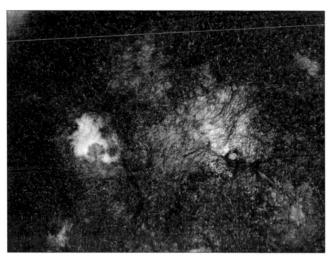

**2.9** Scarring alopecia with hypopigmentation due to previous discoid lupus rash on the scalp (note the patch of hair loss with no signs of new hair growth).

Raynaud's phenomenon is common but usually milder than in systemic sclerosis (**2.10A, B**). However it can be associated with severe digital ischaemia and the development of gangrene (**2.11A, B**). Raynaud's phenomenon may be hard to identify in dark skin unless there is sparing of some fingers (**2.12**). Vasculitic skin rashes may occur on the hands (**2.13A, B**) or the feet (**2.13C, D**) and are less common than the maculopapular rashes of lupus (**2.14**). Vasculitic lesions may progress to frank ulceration (**2.15**) with the risk of secondary infection. Although blistering lesions can occur in lupus patients, shingles due to herpes zoster is more common, especially in

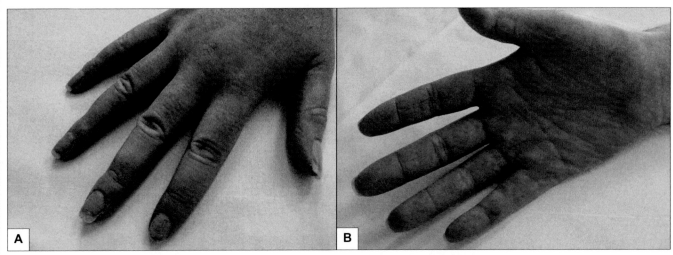

**2.10A, B**: Raynaud's phenomenon may not look severe (right hand dorsal and palmar surfaces).

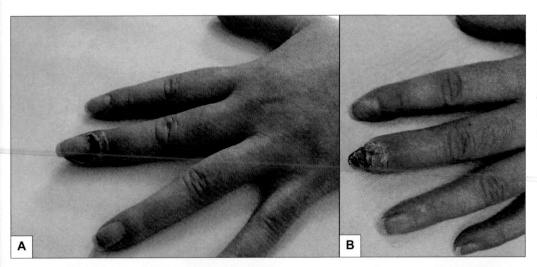

**2.11A, B**: Raynaud's phenomenon progressed to digital ischaemia and gangrene in the left hand of the lupus patient shown in Figure **2.10**.

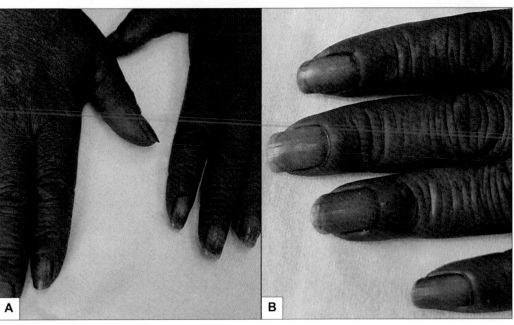

**2.12A, B**: Raynaud's phenomenon may affect some fingers and spare others, making it easier to identify in the affected fingers even if the skin is dark.

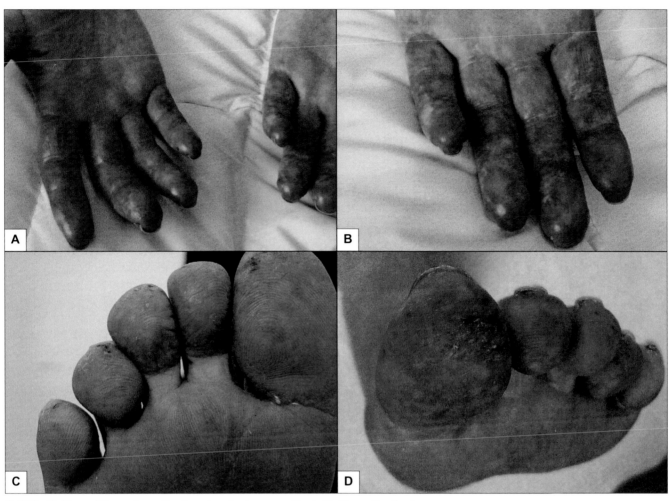

**2.13A, B**: Vasculitic rash on the hands of a lupus patient; **C, D**: on the feet.

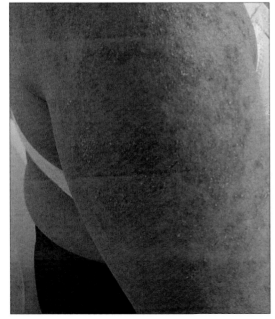

**2.14** Maculopapular rash on the arm due to lupus.

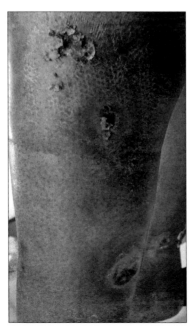

**2.15** Vasculitic ulcers on the legs of a patient with lupus.

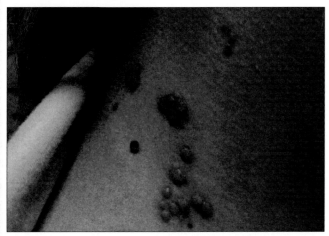

**2.16** Herpes zoster may cause shingles, a blistering rash, particularly in immunosuppressed patients with lupus.

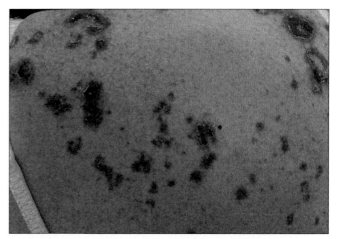

**2.17** Infected maculopapular rash in a patient on high-dose steroids for lupus flare with swabs that grew *Staphylococcus aureus*.

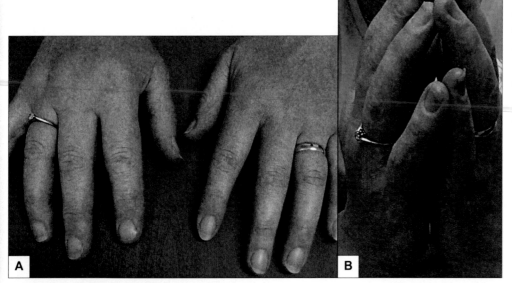

**2.18A, B**: Severe lupus inflammatory arthritis causing swelling in the wrists, metacarpo-phalangeal and proximal interphalangeal joints that limits the patient from putting her hands in the prayer position.

A

B

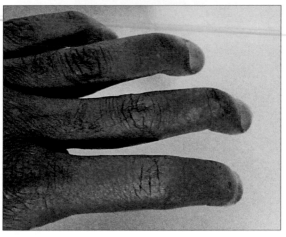

**2.19** Early Jaccoud's arthropathy with a reducible swan neck deformity causing hyperflexion of the distal interphalangeal joint and hyperextension of the proximal interphalangeal joint.

patients on immunosuppressants (**2.16**). Maculopapular rashes may also become infected (**2.17**). Mucocutaneous features are more prominent in Asians and Caucasians, and are less common in people of African descent. With increasing age, secondary Sjögren's syndrome becomes more common with oral and ocular dryness due to mucosal gland destruction as in primary Sjögren's syndrome, though salivary and lacrimal gland swelling is not seen.

## Musculoskeletal manifestations

Generalized inflammatory joint pain (arthralgia) with early morning stiffness or gelling after a period of rest is very common. A nonerosive arthritis with joint tenderness and swelling may develop (**2.18A, B**). Deformities are unusual but may occur due to ligamentous laxity (Jaccoud's arthropathy; **2.19**), in contrast to those of rheumatoid arthritis where the deformities are associated with joint erosions. It should be noted that patients with lupus may develop osteoarthritis as they get older. Heberden's nodes at the distal interphalangeal joints (**2.20A, B**) and Bouchard nodes at the proximal interphalangeal joints due to osteophytes in osteoarthritis should not be confused with acute synovitis due to a lupus flare (**2.21**).

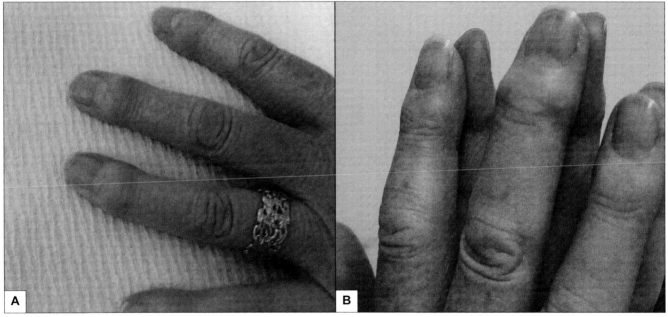

**2.20A, B**: Osteoarthritis with osteophytes causing bony swelling of the distal interphalangeal joints (Heberden's nodes) in a patient with lupus.

**2.21** Synovial swelling of the proximal interphalangeal joints due to lupus flare.

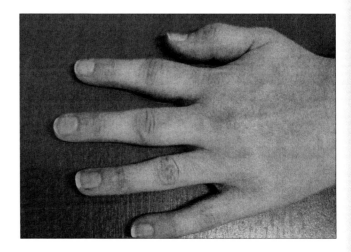

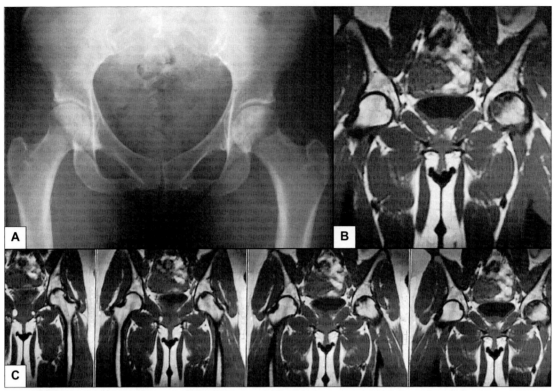

**2.22A**: Plain X-ray showing avascular necrosis of the left hip, which is seen more clearly to affect at least 50% of the femoral head on MR scans (**B, C**).

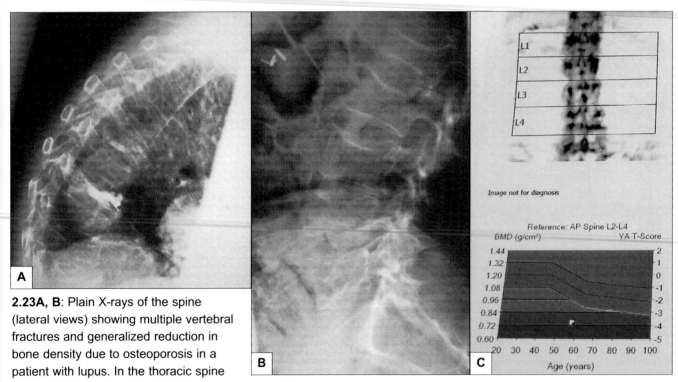

**2.23A, B**: Plain X-rays of the spine (lateral views) showing multiple vertebral fractures and generalized reduction in bone density due to osteoporosis in a patient with lupus. In the thoracic spine (**A**) there are fractures at T7, T10, and T11 and at T9 there is increased density where a vertebroplasty has been performed. In (**B**) there are biconcave wedge fractures at all levels in the lumbar spine (most severe at L1) in this same patient. Very low bone mineral density is confirmed on DEXA scan with a young adult T score of -3.7, well below the age related mean BMD shown by the line in the middle of the blue shading in (**C**).

Myalgia with muscle stiffness is common but a true inflammatory myositis occurs in less than 10% of patients. It should be noted that a myopathy may occur secondary to corticosteroids, antimalarials, or lipid lowering agents. Avascular necrosis or infection (aseptic arthritis) should be suspected if a patient develops sudden onset, severe pain in a single joint. Plain X-ray (**2.22A**) is not as good as MR scan for assessing severity (**2.22B, C**). Patients with SLE who are on steroids, especially those in the postmenopausal age range, are at increased risk for osteoporotic fractures from minimal or no trauma. Plain X-rays (**2.23A–C**) will show insufficiency fractures and wedge fractures but MR

scans are required if there is any concern about compression of the spinal cord or spinal nerve roots (**2.24A, B**).

### Respiratory features

Pain on deep inspiration due to pleurisy is common in SLE. Patients may have signs of pleural rub or small effusion (**2.25A, B**) or not (**2.25C**). Less common manifestations are lupus pneumonitis leading to pulmonary fibrosis (**2.26A, B**), pulmonary haemorrhage, and pulmonary embolism. Pulmonary haemorrhage may develop suddenly and has a high mortality.

**2.24A, B**: Lateral views of the MR scan of the spine of the patient shown in Figures **2.23A–C** showing widespread vertebral fractures in the thoracic (**A**) and lumbar spine (**B**) that spare the cervical spine and do not cause impingement of the spinal cord at any level.

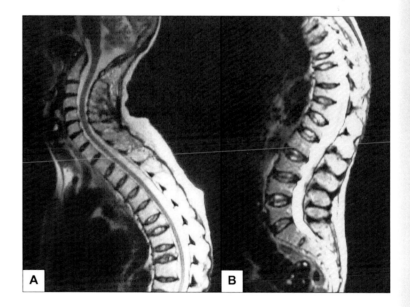

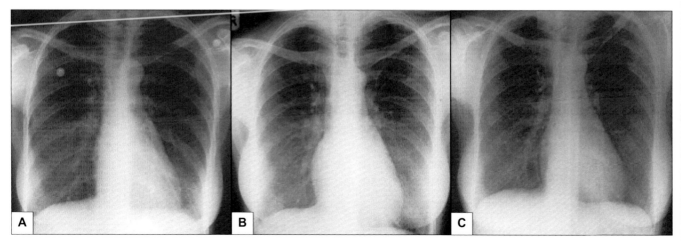

**2.25A, B**: Blunting of the costophrenic angles due to small pleural effusions in a lupus patient with pleuritic chest pain first on the left (**A**), later on the right (**B**); **C**: an episode of pain without any effusions in the same patient.

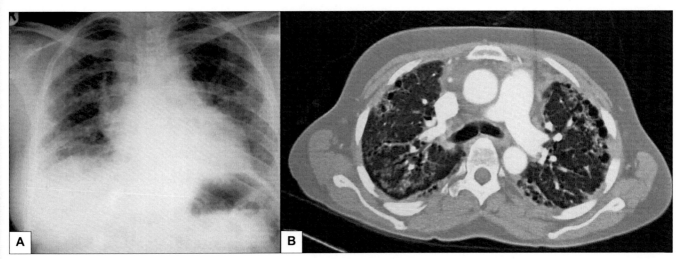

**2.26A, B**: Chest X-ray of the lungs (**A**) and CT pulmonary angiogram (**B**) from a lupus patient who became acutely short of breath. There is evidence of shrinking lung syndrome and severe pulmonary fibrosis on the plain X-ray (**A**). On the CT scan (**B**) there are no filling defects in the vasculature to suggest pulmonary emboli but there are some small peripheral lung cysts, as well as fibrotic change and some patchy air space shadowing suggesting infection.

## Cardiovascular features

The most common cardiovascular presentation of lupus is chest pain that is worse lying down due to pericarditis. This may be associated with small pericardial effusion but tamponade is rare. Myocarditis is much less common and presents with arrhythmias or heart failure. Mitral valve prolapse is found in about 10% of patients at echocardiography but is usually clinically silent. Aseptic endocarditis may occur and usually affects the mitral or aortic valves. Some studies suggest that this is more common in patients with APS. Pulmonary hypertension is associated with a poor prognosis, especially in pregnancy but is fortunately uncommon, occurring in less than 10% of patients. Predisposing factors to pulmonary hypertension include lung fibrosis and previous pulmonary embolism. Coronary artery disease is occasionally caused by vasculitis, but more often results from premature atherosclerosis and is an important cause of death in lupus patients.

## Neuropsychiatric features

SLE may affect the central and peripheral nervous systems (*Tables 2.12, 2.13*). The most common central nervous system manifestations are headache, cerebrovascular accidents, seizures, and aseptic meningitis. Antiphospholipid antibodies (anti-cardiolipin antibodies and/or lupus anticoagulant) may be associated with cerebrovascular accidents (**2.27**), seizures, and chorea. Mood disorders such as depression and headaches are more often due to nonlupus causes including psychosocial issues, sepsis, drugs, uraemia, severe hypertension, hypo-

| Table 2.12 Central nervous system manifestations in systemic lupus erythematosus |
| --- |
| Acute confusional state |
| Aseptic meningitis |
| Anxiety disorder |
| Cerebrovascular disease |
| Cognitive dysfunction |
| Demyelinating syndrome |
| Headache (including benign intracranial hypertension) |
| Mood disorder |
| Movement disorders (including chorea) |
| Myelopathy |
| Psychosis |
| Seizure disorders |

thyroidism, and metabolic disorders. Steroids are often blamed for inducing psychosis, but this is rare with doses equivalent to 30 mg prednisolone daily or less, and if any doubt exists, patients should be given more, not less, steroid, particularly if there is active lupus in other systems and an antipsychotic agent.

**Table 2.13 Peripheral nervous system manifestations in systemic lupus erythematosus**

Acute inflammatory demyelinating polyradiculoneuropathy (Guillain–Barré syndrome)

Autonomic disorder

Mononeuropathy (single or multiplex)

Myasthenia gravis

Neuropathy, cranial

Plexopathy

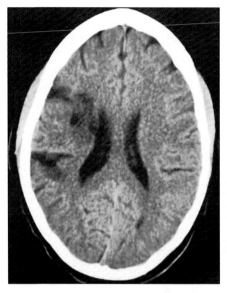

**2.27** CT brain scan of a patient with an infarct in the right middle cerebral artery territory due to thrombosis.

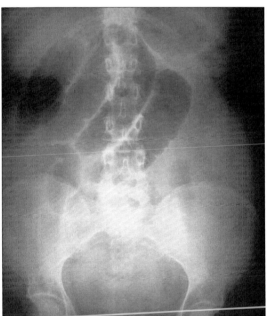

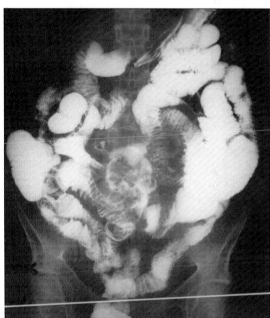

**2.28** Plain X-ray of the abdomen in a patient with subacute bowel obstruction due to lupus.

**2.29** Barium follow-through study in the patient in **2.28** with subacute bowel obstruction showing luminal narrowing, circular fold thickening, irregular with speculation, stacked coin sign, and thumb-printing.

**2.30** CT scan of the abdomen showing dilation, bowel wall thickening with abnormal enhancement and ascites in the lupus patient shown in Figures **2.28**, **2.29**.

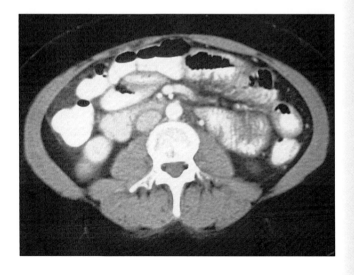

### Gastrointestinal manifestations

Nausea is the most common manifestation. Vomiting is less common but may occur with abdominal pain. Diarrhoea is not common but may occur with active disease, especially protein-losing enteropathy. Vomiting with abdominal pain and constipation are important signs of mesenteric vasculitis but these features can occur in patients with subacute bowel obstruction (**2.28–2.30**) or aseptic

**Table 2.14 Simplified version of the International Society of Nephrology/Renal Pathology Society classification of lupus nephritis (see Figures 2.31–2.34)**

**Class I** — ***Minimal mesangial lupus nephritis***
Normal at light microscopy.
Mesangial deposits on immunofluorescence

**Class II** — ***Mesangial proliferative lupus nephritis***
Mesangial hypercellularity or expansion with mesangial immune deposits.
Some subepithelial or subendothelial deposits on immunofluorescence or electron microscopy

**Class III** — ***Focal lupus nephritis***
Involves <50% glomeruli. Active or inactive lesions typically with subendothelial deposits

**Class IV** — ***Diffuse lupus nephritis***
Involves >50% glomeruli. Active or inactive diffuse, segmental, or global endo- or extracapillary glomerulonephritis. Typically with subendothelial deposits. Divided into diffuse segmental when <50% of involved glomeruli have segmental lesions and diffuse global when >50% of involved glomeruli have global lesions

**Class V** — ***Membranous lupus nephritis***
Global or segmental subepithelial immune deposits by light microscopy and immunofluorescence or electron microscopy, with or without mesangial changes.
Class V lupus nephritis may occur in combination with class III or class IV disease, in which case both are diagnosed.
Class V disease may show advanced sclerosis

**Class VI** — ***Advanced sclerosis lupus nephritis***
>90% of glomeruli globally sclerosed without residual activity

peritonitis. It is essential to exclude or treat infection in patients with these conditions. They usually have other signs of active disease clinically and/or serologically and improve with high-dose steroid therapy. although cyclophosphamide may be required as well. Other abdominal manifestations include hepatitis, sclerosing cholangitis, pancreatitis, and ascites. In all cases the differential diagnosis is infection (viral or bacterial) that should be actively sought before starting treatment with immunosuppressive agents.

### Renal involvement

In the early and most reversible phase of nephritis, lupus patients do not get any symptoms from their kidneys so the urine has to be assessed for protein, cells, and casts. Blood pressure should also be monitored as hypertension is common in lupus nephritis. In patients with membranous nephropathy frank nephrotic syndrome may develop with proteinuria >3.5 g per day, hypoalbuminaemia, hypertension, and oedema. Patients with proteinuria >0.5 g in 24 hours (or a protein:creatinine ratio of >50 mg/mmol) and red cells or casts in the urine should undergo renal biopsy. In the absence of red cells and casts, renal biopsy is not usually performed until the proteinuria level is >1 g in 24 hours or the protein:creatinine ratio is >100 mg/mmol. Renal biopsy is important as patients may have proliferative glomerulonephritis, membranous nephropathy, thrombotic microangiopathy (associated with APS), or a combination of features. In 2003 a revised method for classifying renal biopsies was published by the International Society of Nephrology and the Renal Pathology Society for the classification of lupus nephritis (*Table 2.14*). Examples of the histology seen in proliferative (classes II, III, and IV) and in membranous (class V) glomerulonephritis are shown in Figures **2.31–2.34**. Management depends on the histology and is designed to prevent renal failure.

### Ophthalmic manifestations

The most common causes of red eye in lupus are episcleritis (**2.35A**) and sicca (dry eye) due to secondary Sjögren's syndrome that can be treated just with artificial tear drops. More serious but rare is anterior uveitis, which is distinguished symptomatically by pain in the eye and photophobia. If posterior uveitis develops there will be blurring and loss of vision. Scleritis and keratitis are rare (**2.35B**). The most serious and most common causes of visual loss are optic neuritis and retinal vasculitis (2.36–2.38). Other causes of visual loss include vaso-occlusive disease affecting retinal or choiroidal vessels and anterior ischaemic optic neuropathy. Rarely orbital inflammation occurs with myositis of the eye muscles causing diplopia and/or proptosis. Urgent assessment by an ophthalmologist is required to determine the correct diagnosis in most cases and to decide if treatment should be with immunosuppressives or antiplatelet drugs or anticoagulation. Sometimes it is difficult to be sure whether the underlying pathology is inflammatory, thrombotic, or both and it is often important to exclude infection.

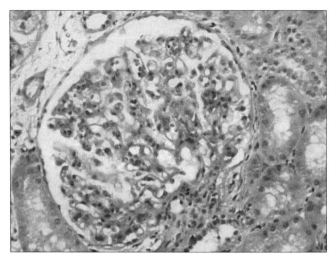

**2.31** Mesangial proliferative glomerulonephritis due to lupus: International Society of Nephrology/Renal Pathology Society (ISN/RPS) class II (see *Table 2.14*).

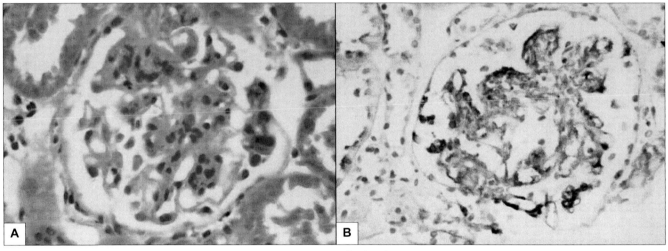

**2.32A, B**: Focal proliferative glomerulonephritis due to lupus: ISN/RPS class III (see *Table 2.14*).

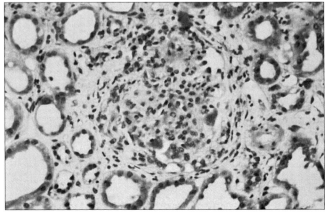

**2.33** Diffuse proliferative glomerulonephritis due to lupus: ISN/RPS class IV (see *Table 2.14*).

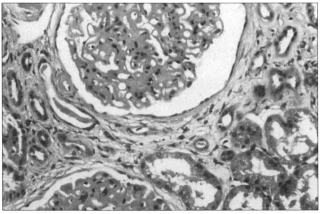

**2.34** Membranous proliferative glomerulonephritis due to lupus: ISN/RPS class V (see *Table 2.14*).

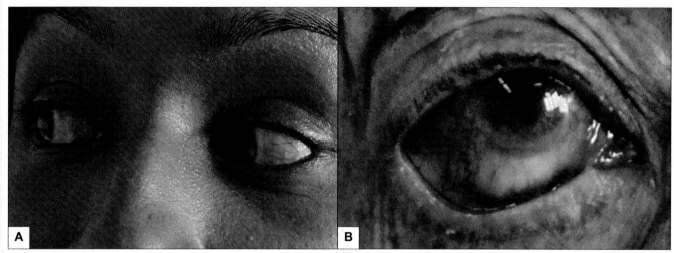

**2.35A**: Episcleritis affecting both eyes; **B**: keratitis affecting the right eye.

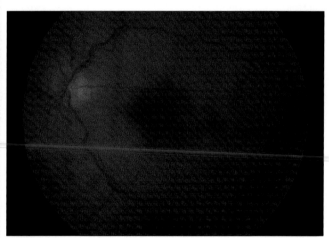

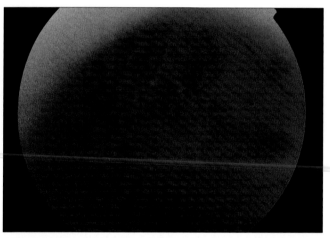

**2.36** Right fundus showing swollen optic disc, elevation and haemorrhage at macula, some superficial retinal haemorrhages with some peripheral haemorrhages that look like Roth spots due to retinal vasculitis in a lupus patient.

**2.37** Peripheral, superficial retinal haemorrhages and exudates in a lupus patient with retinal vasculitis.

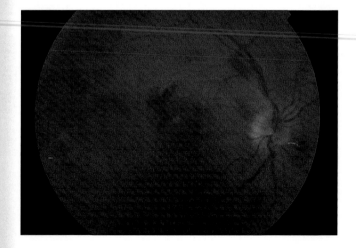

**2.38** Left fundus showing slightly swollen optic disc, elevation and haemorrhage at macula, some superficial retinal haemorrhages with some peripheral haemorrhages that look like Roth spots.

### Haematological features

Low white cell counts are found in some untreated lupus patients. The most typical feature of lupus is lymphopenia, which is found in over 90% of patients. The lymphopenia is antibody mediated. Neutropenia is much more uncommon and rarely associated with infection, though it is found most often in patients of Afro-Caribbean or African-American ethnicity, in whom mild neutropenia is common even in healthy people.

The least common but most significant haematological manifestation is antibody-mediated thrombocytopenia, which can cause bleeding with platelet counts below $50 \times 10^9/l$, though patients with APS often have platelet counts of about $70-90 \times 10^9/l$ and this is associated with an increased risk of thrombosis.

Autoimmune haemolytic anaemia may also occur in lupus but is less common than an anaemia of chronic disease. Haemolysis may be identified by a positive Coombs' test, low haptoglobins, increased reticulocyte count, and/or raised nonconjugated bilirubin. Patients with an anaemia of chronic disease need to be distinguished from those with iron deficiency anaemia due to dietary deficiency and/or blood loss from the gut due to drugs or occasionally bowel involvement by the disease.

### Obstetric issues

Lupus is not associated with infertility but can be associated with recurrent pregnancy losses, particularly in the second or third trimester due to APS or lupus flare. Secondary APS may also predispose to pre-eclampsia and thrombosis in the mother during pregnancy. The mother with lupus should be monitored for intrauterine growth restriction due to placental insufficiency and pre-eclampsia in a specialist unit. Planned early delivery is often required. For mothers with anti-Ro and anti-La antibodies fetal heart rate monitoring should start at 16 weeks' gestation. The risk of congenital heart block in these fetuses is about 1% but the risk of neonatal lupus syndrome with photosensitive rash and sometimes liver dysfunction is about 5%.

### Immunological abnormalities: autoantibodies and complement

Lupus is associated with the development of autoantibodies that precede the onset of clinical features. The most typical but nonspecific antibodies are anti-nuclear antibodies (ANAs), which occur in over 95% of patients. These ANAs can occur in other connective tissue diseases, para-neoplastic conditions, and infections such as glandular fever. More specific antibodies that are not found in other conditions are anti-double stranded DNA antibodies that can be used for diagnosis and monitoring of the disease and anti-Smith (anti-Sm) antibodies. Anti-Sm antibodies are part of a group of antibodies that recognize extractable nuclear antigens (anti-ENA antibodies). This anti-ENA group includes anti-Ro and anti-La antibodies that also occur in primary Sjögren's syndrome and that predispose to neonatal lupus syndrome. Anti-RNP antibodies are part of this group and can also occur in overlap syndromes such as mixed connective tissue disease. Mixed connective tissue disease has features of lupus, systemic sclerosis, and autoimmune myositis.

There are many autoantibodies in lupus and only a few are tested for in patients. The generalized overactivity of plasma cells in producing antibodies is indicated by the increase in gamma-globulins on serum electrophoresis and by increased levels of total immunoglobulin-G (IgG) in many lupus patients, though levels are not as high as those that can be seen in primary Sjögren's syndrome. About 5% of lupus patients have low levels of IgA that may act as a predisposing factor to lupus by increasing the risk of infection through mucosal surfaces, though these patients do not necessarily manifest a higher rate of infection than other lupus patients.

Complement activation occurs in response to the formation of immune complexes when autoantibodies bind to their target antigens. Active disease, particularly lupus nephritis and vasculitis, may be associated with low circulating levels of complements C3 and C4, and increased levels of complement degradation products such as C3d. Thus complement levels may be used to monitor disease activity.

## Diagnosis and differential diagnosis

The diagnosis of lupus is made by identifying a multisystem disease with typical features of lupus associated with the production of autoantibodies. The American College of Rheumatology (formerly the American Rheumatism Association) classification criteria for SLE are often used as diagnostic criteria (*Table 2.10*). They were not designed for this purpose but rather to provide criteria for patients going into clinical trials or long-term outcome studies. To fulfil these criteria patients should have four of the 11 criteria listed in *Table 2.10* at any point in time. It should be noted that these criteria do not include many features of lupus and allow patients to be classified even if they have not had autoantibodies documented. In clinical practice it is best not to make the diagnosis of lupus without some evidence of relevant autoantibody formation. For example, a patient with malar rash, diffuse alopecia, arthritis, digital vasculitis, and a positive ANA with low complements would be diagnosed as having SLE despite only having three classification criteria whereas a patient with photosensitivity, oral ulcers, arthritis, no autoantibodies, and normal complement levels would not be. Similarly a patient with arthritis and classical biopsy-proven class IV glomerulonephritis and positive ANA would be diagnosed as having SLE but not a patient with epilepsy, thrombocytopenia, anti-cardiolipin antibodies, and pleurisy due to a pulmonary embolus, in whom the more appropriate diagnosis would be APS. Conditions that may need to be considered in the differential diagnosis of lupus are listed in *Table 2.15*.

## Table 2.15 Differential diagnosis of lupus

### *Rheumatological conditions*

Rheumatoid arthritis

Primary Sjögren's syndrome

Dermatomyositis

Systemic sclerosis

### *Nonrheumatological conditions*

Infection

Lymphoma

Other malignancies

Porphyria

Discoid rash without systemic disease

# Monitoring disease activity and distinguishing damage

Patients with lupus have lifelong disease and should be monitored at intervals depending on their disease manifestations, blood results, and therapy. Patients with very active disease requiring high-dose steroids and other immunosuppressants are usually seen at least monthly and may require blood tests 2-weekly. For patients with renal involvement assessment will need to be at least 3-monthly even when they appear to have improved and more frequently if immunosuppressive therapy is being reduced or has been discontinued. Patients that appear clinically stable but have rising titres of anti-dsDNA antibodies and/or low complement levels may need to be seen more frequently, as these tests suggest that a lupus flare may occur though it is hard to predict when. Assessment of patients should include a review of all systems including urinalysis, blood pressure, and measures of renal function to assess renal involvement, as well as full blood count and measurement of anti-dsDNA antibodies, C3, and C4. If proteinuria is detected, quantification should occur using a timed urine collection (usually 12 or 24 hours) or measurement of protein:creatinine ratio (in some places albumin:creatinine ratio). Microscopy of the urine is required to identify red and white cells and casts and a sample should be sent for culture to exclude infection.

It is important to distinguish irreversible damage (scarring) due to the disease from disease activity and to identify comorbid conditions such as infection, malignancy, and drug side-effects. It should be noted that malignancy is more common in lupus patients than expected, especially lymphoma. Lung cancer is increased particularly in patients that smoke. A summary of complications that can occur in lupus patients due to the disease or its treatment that are recorded by the Systemic Lupus International Collaborating Clinics/American College of Rheumatology Damage Index is given in *Table 2.16*. For the purposes of the index damage is said to have occurred when a feature appears after the onset of lupus and persists for at least 6 months, or is associated with a classical scar such as myocardial infarction, in which case it can be recorded immediately (see items qualified by the term 'ever' in *Table 2.16*).

**Table 2.16 Systemic Lupus International Collaborating Clinics/American College of Rheumatology Damage Index for patients with lupus**

| Item | Score | Item | Score |
|------|-------|------|-------|
| *Ocular (either eye, by clinical assessment)* | | *Peripheral vascular* | |
| Any cataract ever | 0, 1 | Claudication for 6 months | 0, 1 |
| Retinal change OR optic atrophy | 0, 1 | Minor tissue loss (pulp space) | 0, 1 |
| | | Significant tissue loss ever (e.g. loss of digit or limb) (score 2 if >1 site) | 0, 1, 2 |
| *Neuropsychiatric* | | Venous thrombosis with swelling, ulceration OR venous stasis | 0, 1 |
| Cognitive impairment (e.g. memory deficit, difficulty with calculation, poor concentration, difficulty in spoken or written language, impaired performance level) | | | |
| | | *Gastrointestinal* | |
| | | Infarction or resection of bowel below duodenum, spleen, liver or gall bladder ever, for any cause (score 2 if >1 site) | 0, 1, 2 |
| OR Major psychosis | 0, 1 | Mesenteric insufficiency | 0, 1 |
| Seizures requiring therapy for 6 months | 0, 1 | Chronic peritonitis | 0, 1 |
| Cerebrovascular accident ever (score 2 if >1) | 0, 1, 2 | Stricture OR upper gastrointestinal tract surgery ever | 0, 1 |
| Cranial or peripheral neuropathy (excluding optic) | 0, 1 | Chronic pancreatitis | 0, 1 |
| Transverse myelitis | 0, 1 | | |
| | | *Musculoskeletal* | |
| *Renal* | | Muscle atrophy or weakness | 0, 1 |
| Estimated or measured glomerular filtration rate <50% | 0, 1 | Deforming or erosive arthritis (including reducible deformities, excluding avascular necrosis) | 0, 1 |
| Proteinuria >3.5 g/24 h OR | 0, 1 OR | | |
| End-stage renal disease (regardless of dialysis or transplantation) | 3 | Osteoporosis with fracture or vertebral collapse (excluding avascular necrosis) | 0, 1 |
| | | Avascular necrosis (score 2 if >1) | 0, 1, 2 |
| *Pulmonary* | | Osteomyelitis | 0, 1 |
| Pulmonary hypertension (right ventricular prominence, or loud P2) | 0, 1 | Tendon rupture | 0, 1 |
| Pulmonary fibrosis (physical and radiograph) | 0, 1 | *Skin* | |
| Shrinking lung (radiograph) | 0, 1 | Scarring chronic alopecia | 0, 1 |
| Pleural fibrosis (radiograph) | 0, 1 | Extensive scarring or panniculum other than scalp and pulp space | 0, 1 |
| Pulmonary infarction (radiograph) | 0, 1 | Skin ulceration (excluding thrombosis for >6 months) | 0, 1 |
| *Cardiovascular* | | | |
| Angina OR coronary artery bypass | 0, 1 | *Premature gonadal failure* | |
| Myocardial infarction ever (score 2 if >1) | 0, 1, 2 | *Diabetes* (regardless of treatment) | 0, 1 |
| Cardiomyopathy (ventricular dysfunction) | 0, 1 | *Malignancy* (exclude dysplasia) (score 2 if >1 site) | 0, 1, 2 |
| Valvular disease (diastolic murmur, or systolic murmur >3/6) | 0, 1 | | |
| Pericarditis for 6 months OR pericardiectomy | 0, 1 | | |

Damage (nonreversible change, not related to active inflammation) occurring since onset of lupus, ascertained by clinical assessment and present for at least 6 months unless otherwise stated. Repeat episodes must occur at least 6 months apart to score 2; the same lesion cannot be scored twice

# Principles of management of systemic lupus erythematosus

## Treatment of nonrenal manifestations

Patients with lupus should be advised to avoid exposure to sunlight, to use sunblocks effective against UVA and UVB, and to address lifestyle issues. Hydroxychloroquine (HCQ) is traditionally used to treat joint and skin manifestations with or without corticosteroids locally, orally, or by intramuscular or intravenous injection, depending on the severity of the lupus activity (*Table 2.17*). Evidence is accumulating that HCQ has several beneficial effects beyond controlling joint and skin disease: it seems to protect against thrombotic events, improves lipid profiles, reduces the risk of damage accrual in SLE, and has been shown to have a protective effect on survival. HCQ can be continued in pregnancy and lactation without fetal or neonatal toxicity.

If HCQ is not sufficient or is not tolerated, methotrexate (MTX) may be considered, as it has been shown to reduce arthritis, skin manifestations, and disease activity scores as well as allowing efficient steroid reduction in a randomized controlled trial. However, MTX is contraindicated in women planning pregnancy and during pregnancy and breast-feeding as it causes congenital abnormalities. Corticosteroids in combination with azathioprine (AZA) should be considered if HCQ is not sufficient for women planning pregnancy and in those with more severe organ involvement, but other immunosuppressants such as ciclosporin, lefluonamide, or mycophenolate mofetil (MMF) can be considered in women who are not planning pregnancy and do not respond to steroids, HCQ, and AZA (*Table 2.18*). For organ-threatening disease with vasculitis and major nervous system involvement intravenous corticosteroids may be considered as an alternative to high-dose oral corticosteroids, and cyclophosphamide or MMF is usually given as well, as described below for proliferative glomerulonephritis (*Table 2.19*).

## Treatment of lupus nephritis

The classical treatment still is the administration of high-dose corticosteroids and intravenous (IV) cyclophosphamide (CYC) as an intermittent bolus or pulse therapy. Randomized controlled studies showed that the addition of an immunosuppressant, especially CYC, to corticosteroids was more effective in lupus nephritis than corticosteroids alone. Over the years, treatment regimens have been modified towards shorter periods and lower doses of CYC and more rapid steroid reduction. The most widely used National Institutes of Health (NIH) therapy regimen comprises IV CYC once per month for 6 months followed by a bolus once every 3 months for up to 2 years. The European Lupus Trials have demonstrated that 'low-dose CYC' of 500 mg every 2 weeks on six occasions, then AZA was as efficacious as the NIH protocol that used higher doses of CYC with regard to the development of end-stage renal failure. Recent studies have shown equal efficacy and less toxicity for MMF compared to oral and intravenous bolus CYC. MMF is increasingly being used as

**Table 2.17 Treatment of mild SLE**

| System | Examples of manifestations | Treatment of acute flare may include any of the following: | Maintenance therapy to prevent flare may include any of the following: |
|---|---|---|---|
| Mucocutaneous | Nonvasculitic localized rashes Mucosal ulceration Alopecia: diffuse or mild patchy loss | Local (to skin or mucous membranes or intra-articular) corticosteroids | Hydroxychloroquine (<6.5 mg/kg/day) |
| Musculoskeletal | Arthralgia/mild or intermittent arthritis &/or myalgia | Low-dose oral corticosteroids (e.g. 5–10 mg prednisolone) | Low-dose oral corticosteroids (e.g. 5–10 mg prednisolone) |
| Cardiorespiratory | Pleuritic or pericardial pain without rub or effusion | NSAIDs short term | |

it does not cause infertility. CYC should be administered for as short a time as possible because of ovarian or testicular toxicity and the risk of infection, usually 3–6 months, and is then replaced by an alternative. There is evidence to support AZA, MMF, or ciclosporin A as maintenance therapy in SLE nephritis.

### Table 2.18 Treatment of moderate SLE

| System | Examples of manifestations | Treatment of acute flare may include any of the following: | Maintenance therapy to prevent flare may include any of the following: |
|---|---|---|---|
| Mucocutaneous | Extensive maculopapular or discoid or blistering rash<br>Vasculitic rash<br>Erythema nodosum or localized panniculitis<br>Severe patchy alopecia +/- scarring | Moderate-dose corticosteroids (e.g. starting at ≤0.5 mg/kg/day prednisolone) | Reduce prednisolone slowly to 0.1 mg/kg/day |
| Musculoskeletal | Persistent arthritis with swelling and/or loss of function | IM or IV dose of methylprednisolone (e.g. 100–500 mg) | Hydroxychloroquine (≤6.5 mg/kg/day) |
| Cardiorespiratory | Pleurisy or pericarditis with rub or small effusion | Start or increase AZA, OR MTX, OR ciclosporin, OR lefluonamide | Maintenance dose of AZA (1–2 mg/kg/day), OR MTX (≤25 mg/week), OR ciclosporin (≤2.5 mg/kg/day), OR lefluonamide (20 mg/day) |
| Gastrointestinal | Abdominal serositis | | |

### Table 2.19 Treatment of severe SLE

| System | Examples of manifestations | Treatment of acute flare may include any of the following: | Maintenance therapy to prevent flare may include any of the following: |
|---|---|---|---|
| Mucocutaneous | Extensive vasculitic rash with ulceration or infarction or extensive panniculitis | High-dose corticosteroids (e.g. starting at ≤0.75–1.0 mg/kg/day prednisolone) | Reduce prednisolone slowly to 0.1 mg/kg/day |
| Musculoskeletal | Persistent polyarthritis with marked loss of function | IV doses of methylprednisolone (e.g. 500 mg × 3) | Hydroxychloroquine (≤6.5 mg/kg/day) |

*Continued overleaf*

**Table 2.19** *Continued*

| System | Examples of manifestations | Treatment of acute flare may include any of the following: | Maintenance therapy to prevent flare may include any of the following: |
| --- | --- | --- | --- |
| Cardiorespiratory | Pleurisy or pericarditis with large effusions or tamponade<br>Lupus pneumonitis | Start or increase cyclophosphamide IV pulses (2–4 weekly for 3–6 months) OR oral MMF or IV rituximab (e.g. 1000 mg × 2 +/- IV cyclophosphamide 2 doses) | Maintenance dose of AZA (1–2 mg/kg/day), OR MTX (≤25 mg/week), OR ciclosporin (≤2.5 mg/kg/day), OR lefluonamide (20 mg/day), OR MMF (2–3 g/day), OR IV cyclophosphamide pulses 3 monthly |
| Gastrointestinal | Gut vasculitis or subacute intestinal obstruction or lupus pancreatitis | | |
| Genitourinary | Proliferative glomerulonephritis<br>Membranous glomerulonephritis with nephritic syndrome<br>Lupus cystitis with or without ureteric involvement | | |

## 'Biologics' in SLE

Case reports and case series suggested a beneficial effect in SLE of rituximab, a monoclonal CD20-antibody approved for the use in B cell lymphoma. Rituximab showed a significant improvement in SLAM (systemic lupus activity measure) score in a phase I/II dose escalation study, and may also have a benefit in disease refractory to all other treatments. Recently, belimumab has demonstrated effectiveness in lupus trials and is licensed for lupus in USA and Europe.

TNF-antagonists have not been used routinely in SLE, as they may induce lupus-like disease. However, there is now some evidence that short courses of TNF-antagonists may be effective in SLE including nephritis, as shown in a small open-label study.

## Further reading

D'Cruz DP, Khamashta MA, Hughes GR (2007). Systemic lupus erythematosus. *Lancet* **369**(9561):587–96.

Gordon C (2011). Assessing disease activity and outcome in SLE. In: *Rheumatology*, 5th edn. MC Hochberg, AJ Silman, JS Smolen, ME Weinblatt, MH Weisman (eds.). Mosby, Philadelphia, ch.130, pp. 1301–6.

Gordon C, Jayne D, Pusey C, *et al.* (2009). European consensus statement on the terminology used in the management of lupus glomerulonephritis. *Lupus* **18**(3):257–63.

Griffiths B, Mosca M, Gordon C (2005). Assessment of patients with systemic lupus erythematosus and the use of lupus disease activity indices. *Best Pract Res Clin Rheumatol* **19**(5):685–708.

Kumar K, Chambers S, Gordon C (2009). Challenges of ethnicity in SLE. *Best Pract Res Clin Rheumatol* **23**(4):549–61.

Amissah-Arthur MB, Gordon C (2010). Contemporary treatment of systemic lupus erythematosus: an update for clinicians. *Therapeutic Advances in Chronic Disease* Nov 1:163–75.

Ruiz-Irastorza G, Khamashta MA (2009). Managing lupus patients during pregnancy. *Best Pract Res Clin Rheumatol* **23**(4):575–82.

Tsokos G, Gordon C, Smolen J (eds.) (2007). *A Companion to Rheumatology: Systemic Lupus Erythematosus.* Mosby/Elsevier Science, Philadelphia.

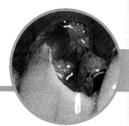

# Chapter 3

# Sjögren's syndrome

*Iona Meryon, Julia U Holle, Wolfgang L Gross, and Caroline Gordon*

## Definition, pathology, and epidemiology

Sjögren's syndrome (SS) is a collection of conditions caused by autoimmune-mediated exocrine dysfunction. It is often associated with other connective tissue diseases, such as rheumatoid arthritis, systemic sclerosis (SSc), systemic lupus erythematosus (SLE), and polymyositis, and termed secondary SS. In the absence of another connective tissue disease, it is classified as primary SS.

SS is characterized by immune-mediated destruction of the exocrine glands. There is a chronic progressive lymphocytic infiltrate, predominantly of the salivary and lacrimal glands, which causes dry eyes and a dry mouth.

SS is one of the most common autoimmune disorders. The population prevalence of the disease ranges from 0.5% to 5%, split equally between primary and secondary disease. Secondary SS complicates one-third of cases of autoimmune rheumatic disease. Eight percent of those with no clinical diagnosis of SS had significant lymphocytic infiltrate at postmortem. It affects nine times more women than men. The commonest time to develop SS is after the menopause. Symptoms of dry eyes and mouth are extremely common, particularly in the elderly. In the absence of a lymphocytic infiltrate or associated connective tissue disease, dry eyes and dry mouth are termed 'sicca', meaning 'dry' in Latin.

## Clinical manifestations and assessment of Sjögren's syndrome

The majority of symptoms relate to salivary and lacrimal dysfunction. Mucosal dryness often predates definitive diagnosis by many years, and symptoms of dry eyes and mouth are under-reported. No difference in presentation has been described when variations in age, sex, and geographical origin are analysed. SS is a multisystem disease, and the extraglandular manifestations are explored in a later section. The most common complaints relate to glandular features, and can be divided into oral and ocular symptoms.

### Ocular symptoms

Inflammatory destruction of the conjunctival epithelium causes reduced secretion of tears and chronic irritation. This is termed keratoconjunctivitis sicca.

The most prominent ocular manifestation of SS is the 'dry eye'. However, the initial symptom is often described as a foreign-body sensation, where the eye feels gritty, as if a grain of sand were irritating it. There may be a heightened sensitivity to irritants, such as contact lenses and smoke. Redness, photophobia, and ocular fatigue are later features, along with complications of persisting dryness, such as corneal abrasions and infections.

Three direct questions are useful as a semiobjective method of defining the symptoms of dry eyes (see *Box 1*).

---

**Box 1: Objective assessment of ocular symptoms**

1 Do you have a recurrent sensation of sand or gravel in the eyes?

2 Have you had persistent troublesome dry eyes daily for more than 3 months?

3 Do you use tear substitutes more than three times daily?

---

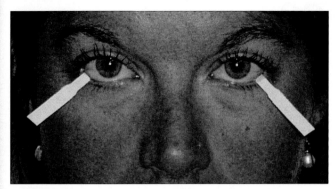

**3.1** Schirmer's test to demonstrate reduced tear production.

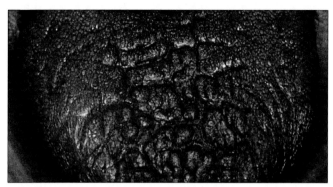

**3.2** Dry tongue and angular cheilosis due to primary SS. (Courtesy of Dr. John Hamburger.)

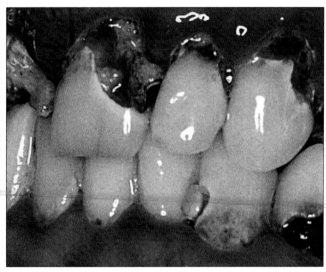

**3.3** Dental caries in SS. (Courtesy of Prof. Iain L.C. Chapple.)

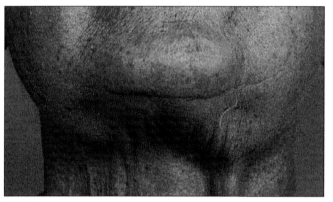

**3.4** Diffuse submandibular gland swelling in primary SS. (Courtesy of Dr. John Hamburger. Reproduced from *Dental Update* [ISSN 0305-5000], with permission of George Warman Publications [UK] Ltd.)

The symptoms of keratoconjunctivitis sicca can be evaluated further. However, these tests lack specificity for SS and must be interpreted in the appropriate clinical context:

### Schirmer's test

This simple test assesses the patient's ability to produce tears, and can be conducted in the out-patient setting. A small strip of sterile filter paper is placed in the lateral third of the eyelid, and in normal individuals the tears moisten over 15 mm of filter paper in 5 minutes. A wetting time of less than 5 mm in 5 minutes is a positive test (**3.1**).

### Rose Bengal stain

Rose Bengal dye binds devitalized and damaged epithelium of the conjunctiva and cornea, which is caused by dehydration in SS. In this test, the dye is administered into each eye before slit-lamp examination. The areas of damaged epithelium become temporarily red-stained and

the degree of such is quantified on the Rose-Bengal Score, where a score of >4 in at least one eye is abnormal. Other dyes may also be used with a correlating scoring system. Punctate ulceration of the cornea is also observed, initially at the inferior corneal margin. A rheumatologist may do a screening examination using the dye with an ophthalmoscope to triage the severity of ocular involvement. Severe keratoconjunctivitis, corneal vasculitis, or abrasions require urgent ophthalmological referral.

### Oral symptoms

Dry mouth (xerostomia) is the principle oral manifestation of SS (**3.2**), and is tolerated less well than the ocular manifestations. The dry mouth causes a burning sensation and altered taste, with difficulty swallowing and speaking. There are many causes of a dry mouth (see *Table 3.1*). Eating can be difficult – the cracker sign describes patients' visible objection to the concept of swallowing a dry cracker

## Table 3.1 Causes of dry mouth

**Iatrogenic**
Drugs, e.g. Anticholinergics
Irradiation: radiotherapy, radio-iodine therapy

**Dehydration**
Primary
Secondary: diabetes mellitus, hypercalcaemia, trauma, diarrhoea

**Viral infections**
Hepatitis C virus, HIV, HTLV

**Psychogenic**

**Congenital defect of salivary gland**

## Table 3.2 Differential diagnosis of parotid swelling

| Unilateral | Bilateral |
|---|---|
| Malignancy | Viral infection: EBV, Coxsackie A, Mumps, CMV, HIV |
| Bacterial infection | Infiltration: sarcoid, amyloid |
| Chronic sialadenitis | Sjögren's syndrome |
| | Metabolic: diabetes, hyperlipoproteinaemias, chronic pancreatitis, cirrhosis |
| Endocrine | Hypogonadism, acromegaly |

without water. They may drink large volumes of fluids to counteract the symptoms, and some patients complain they wake at night needing to drink water.

Xerostomia accelerates dental decay and the resulting caries appears in unusual sites such as the incisors and gingival line (**3.3**). There is an increased risk of salivary calculi formation and oral candidiasis.

The majority of patients with primary SS will experience episodes of parotid and/or submandibular gland swelling (**3.4**). This may begin unilaterally although many become bilateral; parotid enlargement persists in some (*Table 3.2*). This feature is uncommon when the condition is secondary to another connective tissue disease or rheumatoid arthritis. The classification criteria specify three questions to evaluate oral features (see *Box 2*).

Objective evidence of salivary gland involvement is demonstrated with tests used to assess salivary flow and duct structure:

### Unstimulated whole salivary flow
This simple test can be conducted in an out-patient clinic. The patient is asked to hold the mouth open for 1 minute, and pooling of infra-lingual saliva is observed in normal subjects (**3.5**). This can be quantified during an extended period, and is known as sialometry. The patient collects all saliva over a 15-minute period. If there is less than 1.5 ml, it is a positive test. In SS, it is difficult to demonstrate salivary flow from Stensen's duct even when the parotid gland is massaged.

---

**Box 2: Objective assessment of oral symptoms**

1 Have you had a feeling of dry mouth daily for more than 3 months?

2 Do you often need liquids to help swallow food?

3 Have you had recurrent or persistent swelling of the salivary glands as an adult?

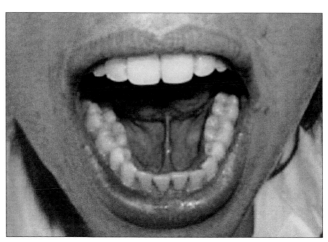

**3.5** Pooling of saliva in a normal individual.

*Parotid sialography*

Contrast is delivered to the parotid gland after retrograde cannulation, and demonstrates dilated ducts (diffuse sialectasis) in the absence of an obstructive cause in SS.

*Salivary scintigraphy*

This radionuclide study demonstrates salivary gland function. Poor uptake of the tracer substance is a very specific feature of SS. Other features include delayed uptake, reduced concentration, or delayed excretion of tracer. There are three notable disadvantages that limit its use. It is an invasive test, it lacks sensitivity as positive results are seen in only one-third of patients, and it can cause episodes of pain and swelling. Both imaging techniques are limited by availability.

## Histopathology

SS is associated with a progressive lymphocytic infiltrate in all the affected organs. The majority of patients have salivary gland involvement, and therefore biopsy of the minor salivary glands is the single most sensitive and specific test used in the diagnosis of SS. The biopsy is usually performed on the buccal mucosa (**3.6**), and must be from tissue that grossly appears normal. The lymphocytic infiltration is quantified by the focus score. This describes the number of aggregations ('foci') of more than 50 lymphocytes and histiocytes in a 4 mm² section of salivary gland tissue. Focus score ≥1 is a positive histological feature of SS (**3.7**). However, cigarette smoking has been reported to lower the focus score.

## Extraglandular disease
*Systemic features*

Although the cardinal feature of SS is lymphocytic infiltration of exocrine glands, the autoimmune response can affect all major organ systems. The syndrome covers a spectrum of clinical manifestations, from features strictly limited to the autoimmune exocrinopathy to a diverse multisystem disease. Systemic features affect one-third of patients with SS – the majority of patients complain of fatigue and episodes of low-grade fever. Extraglandular manifestations are rare when SS is associated with rheumatoid arthritis, but more common when associated with other connective tissue diseases.

The systemic features of SS are attributable either to epithelial lymphocytic infiltration of nonexocrine organs, or wider extraepithelial manifestations. They are associated with the presence of autoantibodies and some of the manifestations may be related to immune complex deposition and complement activation, as in SLE. It is important to identify extraepithelial manifestations of SS as they influence the strategy used in the management of the condition.

*Arthralgia and arthritis*

Arthralgia is the most common extraglandular manifestation. Episodes of nonerosive arthritis are also common, particularly in patients with Raynaud's phenomenon (**3.8A, B** and **3.9**).

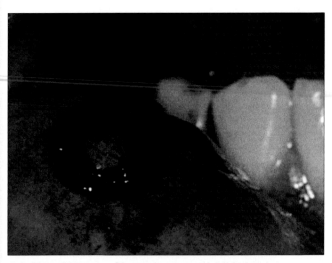

**3.6** Site of biopsy of buccal mucosa labial gland. (Courtesy of Dr. John Hamburger.)

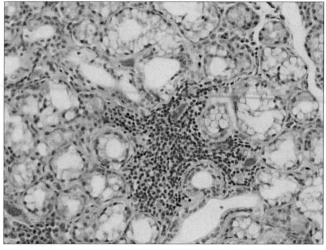

**3.7** Histology of labial gland biopsy in primary SS.

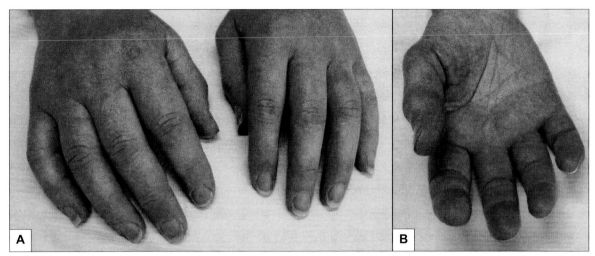

**3.8A**: Raynaud's phenomenon may be subtle on the extensor surface (right first and second digits only) in a patient with arthritis due to primary SS; **B**: Raynaud's phenomenon may be more obvious on the palmar surface (right first and second digits only).

## Myalgia and myositis

Myalgia features in 30% of patients and is attributable to both inflammatory and noninflammatory muscle involvement. Subclinical muscle involvement is common in primary SS, where histological evidence of inflammatory myositis is seen in half of asymptomatic patients.

## Vascular involvement

Raynaud's phenomenon (**3.8A, B**) is seen in one-third of patients and precedes sicca symptoms by several years. It may be the first feature of primary SS. However, Raynaud's phenomenon is also a feature of limited SSc and systemic lupus, therefore it may represent a feature of secondary SS. Anti-centromere antibodies play an important role in distinguishing patients with limited SSc.

## Neurological features

Microvascular involvement causes peripheral and cranial neuropathies. Central nervous system involvement has been described, with clinical signs including hemisensory deficit, hemiparesis, movement disorders, and seizures. However, the actual prevalence and clinical significance of these features are controversial. Sensorineural hearing loss is a feature in up to one-quarter of patients and may be more common in those with anti-cardiolipin antibodies.

## Pulmonary involvement

Respiratory involvement is a common complication of SS, but has subtle symptoms and an insidious clinical course. Dry cough is common and is attributed to dryness of the tracheobronchial mucosa (xerotrachea) and impaired

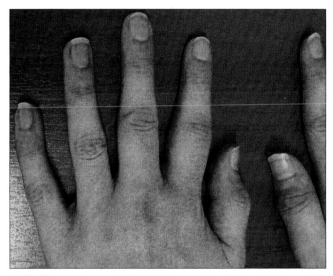

**3.9** Inflammatory arthritis in the proximal interphalangeal joints.

mucociliary clearance. However, inflammatory infiltrate of the small airways and interstitium may sometimes be responsible for respiratory symptoms. Lung disease may occur early in the course of primary SS (particularly if anti-Ro positive) but is not common.

## Gastrointestinal disease

Oropharyngeal dryness is a common cause of dysphagia in SS. It may also result from oesophageal dysmotility in patients with some degree of overlap syndrome and features of SSc. Inflammatory infiltrate of the gastric mucosa has been associated with nausea and epigastric pain. Liver involvement is present in 5% of patients with SS. An important cause is autoimmune cholangitis. Primary biliary cirrhosis is associated with SS; anti-mitochondrial antibodies serve as a sensitive marker of severe underlying liver pathology (see *Table 3.4*). Viral hepatitis can also cause a pseudo-SS (see *Table 3.7*).

### Lymphoproliferative disease

Lymphadenopathy is a common feature in SS and is found in one-third of patients; splenomegaly is found in about 10%. Non-Hodgkin's lymphoma of B cell origin develops in 5% of patients with SS and is considered to be the most important major complication in the natural history of the condition. The interval between the diagnosis of SS and the onset of lymphoma averages 8 years. Prognosis varies with the clinical and histological features (*Table 3.3*). The most common type is MALT (mucosa-associated lymphoid tissue) lymphoma. One study defined the risk of developing lymphoma as 44 times that of the matched populations. Extraglandular features such as vasculitis, fever, lymphadenopathy, and peripheral neuropathies are more common in patients with lymphoma and SS than in patients with only SS.

### Renal disease

Renal impairment affects 5% of patients with SS, and is generally attributable to either tubulointerstitial disease or

| Table 3.3 Poor prognostic features of Sjögren's syndrome-associated lymphoma |
|---|
| Intermediate to high-grade lymphoma |
| B symptoms (fever, night sweats, weight loss) |
| Large tumour diameter (>7 cm) |

glomerular involvement. One-third of patients with SS have abnormal urine acidification, suggesting subclinical infiltration of renal tubules. Renal tubular acidosis is more common in patients who have antibodies to carbonic anhydrase II. Interstitial disease occurs early in the condition and generally follows an indolent course. Glomerulonephritis is a late feature in the disease and is rare but is associated with high morbidity and mortality.

### Autoantibodies

The majority of patients with SS develop autoantibodies during their disease. These play a role in diagnosis and predicting course and severity of disease. The only autoantibodies included in the diagnostic criteria (*Table 3.4*) are anti-SS-A (Anti-Ro) and Anti-SS-B (Anti-La)

### Table 3.4 Relevance of autoantibodies present in Sjögren's syndrome

| Autoantibody | Significance |
|---|---|
| Anti-Ro, anti-La | Diagnosis<br>Extraglandular manifestations (vasculitis, lung)<br>Congenital heart block |
| Rheumatoid factor | Lymphoma evolution<br>Severe salivary gland destruction |
| Cryoglobulins | Lymphoma evolution<br>Severe organ involvement<br>(Poor prognostic indicator) |
| Anti-centromere | Sclerodactyly<br>Raynaud's phenomenon |
| Anti-muscarinic receptor antibodies | Extraglandular muscarinic effects: irritable bladder, heart rate variability, dysphagia |
| Anti-mitochondrial antibodies | Liver involvement, particularly PBC |
| Anti-carbonic anhydrase II antibodies | Distal renal tubular acidosis |

antibodies. However, many others play a role in identifying associated conditions and predicting prognosis and complications.

*Anti-Ro and anti-La antibodies* are seen in 80% and 50% of patients with primary SS, respectively. They correlate with a more severe lymphocytic infiltrate of the salivary glands and have been associated with extraglandular manifestations of disease (such as vasculitis and lung disease). Anti-Ro and anti-La antibiotics are less common in secondary SS. When the condition is associated with rheumatoid arthritis they are present in 10% of patients, and 40% when associated with SLE. In women with anti-Ro and anti-La antibodies, pregnancy may be complicated by neonatal lupus (**3.10**) or congenital heart block, due to transfer of the antibodies across the placenta from week 16 onwards.

*Rheumatoid factor and anti-nuclear antibodies* (ANAs) are found in 90% of patients. Rheumatoid factor correlates with an increased risk of developing lymphoma and severe salivary gland infiltrate. One-fifth of patients with SS have circulating cryoglobulins, which are immunoglobulins that precipitate at temperatures under 37°C and become soluble when rewarmed. The presence of these cryoglobulins at presentation (and particularly a mixed cryoglobulinaemia) correlates closely with development of severe organ involvement and lymphoma and is therefore considered to be a poor prognostic indicator.

*Anti-centromere antibodies* are associated with limited cutaneous sclerosis. Patients with SS who produce anti-centromere antibodies are more likely to have sclerodactyly and Raynaud's phenomenon.

*Anti-muscarinic receptor antibodies.* Glandular secretion occurs via acetylcholine mediation of muscarinic receptors. The M3 subtype of muscarinic receptor accounts for over 90% of these in the parotid gland. Antibodies to an epitope of the M3 receptor (Anti-M3AChR213-228) are found in 90% of patients with primary SS. Anti-muscarinic receptor antibodies are associated with extraglandular manifestations, mostly through muscarinic involvement, such as irritable bladder, heart rate variability, and oesophageal dysmotility.

*Antibodies to carbonic anhydrase II* have been described in SS and correlate with distal tubular acidosis. Anti-mitochondrial antibodies (AMA) are a diagnostic marker of primary biliary cirrhosis (PBC). Although they are an uncommon finding in SS, over 90% of positive AMA have histological evidence of PBC, which develops clinically during 5-year follow-up. Therefore, AMA serves as a sensitive marker of underlying liver pathology in SS and usually represent an asymptomatic stage of PBC.

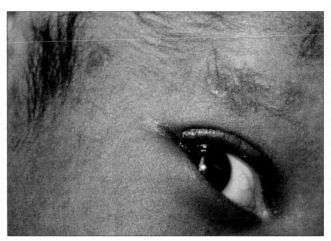

**3.10** Neonatal rash (which looks like subacute cutaneous lupus rash) on the face of a baby born to a mother with primary SS.

## Classification

Many classification criteria have been proposed and revised, leading to significant diagnostic discrepancies. In 2002, an international consensus group collaborated and revised earlier classification sets and produced the criteria currently in use. These provide a validated method for classifying primary and secondary SS, and define specific exclusion criteria (*Table 3.5*).

## Diagnosis and differential diagnosis

The classification criteria of the American–European Consensus Group (*Table 3.5*) are used for diagnosis, although in no way do they negate the role of clinical judgement. Their important role lies in standardizing diagnosis for clinical studies. Diagnosis of primary SS requires evidence of an autoimmune response (either with demonstration of classical histological features or autoantibody production) and lacrimal or salivary involvement. Therefore, diagnosis is made when four of the six criteria are fulfilled, including either positive histopathology or positive immunology results (*Tables 3.5, 3.6*). Secondary SS can only be diagnosed in the context of an established connective tissue disease such as SLE (*Table 3.6*).

There are many conditions without an inflammatory exocrinopathy that mimic SS with symptoms of dryness of the eyes and mouth. However, sicca symptoms accompanied by biopsy evidence of lymphocytic infiltrate of the exocrine glands does not guarantee the underlying diagnosis to be SS. There are several viruses and deposition disorders that have similar symptoms and biopsy findings

**Table 3.5 Revised International Classification Criteria for Sjögren's syndrome**

| | |
|---|---|
| 1 Ocular symptoms | One of:<br>• Recurrent gritty sensation<br>• Daily eye symptoms for 3 months<br>• Use of tear substitute more than three times daily |
| 2 Oral symptoms | One of:<br>• Dry mouth daily for 3 months<br>• Liquids to swallow dry food<br>• Swollen salivary glands |
| 3 Objective evidence of ocular involvement | One of:<br>• Positive Schirmer's test (≤5 mm in 5 mins)<br>• Positive Rose Bengal test (≥4 van Bijstervald's Score) |
| 4 Histopathology | Focal lymphocytic sialadenitis of minor salivary glands AND focus score ≥1 |
| 5 Objective evidence of oral involvement | One of:<br>• Unstimulated whole salivary flow (≤1.5 ml in 15 mins)<br>• Parotid sialography showing diffuse sialectasis (without obstruction)<br>• Salivary scintigraphy showing delayed uptake, reduced concentration, or delayed excretion of tracer |
| 6 Autoantibodies | Anti-Ro (SS-A)<br>Anti-La (SS-B) |

**Table 3.6 Diagnosis of Sjögren's syndrome using the International Consensus criteria**

| *Primary SS* | *Secondary SS* |
|---|---|
| Four of six criteria: including positive histopathology or positive autoantibodies | Established connective tissue disease<br>One sicca symptom (1 or 2)<br>Two positive objective tests (3–5) |

(see *Tables 3.7, 3.8*). Sicca symptoms may also be iatrogenic, secondary to either pharmacological or radiotherapy treatment. These need to be excluded before a diagnosis of SS can be made made.

### HIV

Human immunodeficiency virus (HIV)-positive patients may initially present with sicca symptoms, lympha-denopathy, parotid swelling, and pulmonary involvement. This condition, known as diffuse infiltrative lymphocytosis syndrome (DILS), is seen in 5% of HIV-positive patients, and is more common in young men. Although RF and ANA may be positive, they produce no autoantibodies to Ro (SS-A) and La (SS-B). There is a CD8+ predominant lymphocytic infiltrate on biopsy. It is often associated with the HLA-DR5 autoantigen.

| Table 3.7 Exclusion criteria |
| --- |
| Hepatitis C infection |
| HIV infection |
| Sarcoidosis |
| Lymphoma (predating symptoms) |
| Previous head/neck radiotherapy |
| Graft versus host disease |
| Anticholinergic drugs (symptoms within four times the half-life of the drug) |

| Table 3.8 Conditions causing lymphocytic infiltrate of exocrine glands |
| --- |
| HIV |
| Hepatitis C |
| HTLV-1 virus |
| Sarcoidosis |
| Amyloidosis |
| Haemochromatosis |
| Graft versus host disease |

### Hepatitis C

There is a close relationship between hepatitis C and SS. The virus causes a lymphocytic sialadenitis, and up to three-quarter of hepatitis C-positive patients have clinical and histological features of SS. Histologically, there are less severe lesions and lower focus scores. However, they have a higher prevalence of neurological and liver involvement, cryoglobulinaemia, and hypocomplementaemia, but are less likely to produce autoantibodies to Ro and La (SS-A and SS-B).

### HTLV-1 virus

Human T-lymphotrophic virus type 1 (HTLV-1) infection is endemic in Japan, where a relationship between the infection and SS has been well described. HTLV-1 infects the epithelial cells of the salivary glands, causing a chronic sialadenitis. Clinically and serologically the conditions are identical; however, sialography is often nondiagnostic in HTLV-1 infection.

### Infiltrative disease

Sarcoid can masquerade as SS, with sicca symptoms, systemic features, hypergammaglobulinaemia, and pulmonary involvement. However, on biopsy, noncaseating granulomas confirm the diagnosis of sarcoidosis. Similarly, amyloid infiltration of the salivary glands mimics the oral manifestations of SS, but birefringence and immuno-chemical staining of the biopsy demonstrate typical amyloid changes.

### Haemochromatosis

Sicca features and salivary gland swelling have been described in patients with haemochromatosis. Salivary gland biopsy is useful in identifying these cases, where histological examination reveals iron deposition in the absence of a lymphocytic infiltrate.

### Graft versus host disease

Lymphocytic infiltration of the salivary glands occurs up to 1 year after bone marrow transplantation, and can be associated with positive ANA and smooth muscle antibodies. The graft versus host response causes similar symptoms to SS, which can persist for up to 2 years.

### Other important differential diagnoses

Sicca symptoms are also common in patients with fibromyalgia, depression, and bulimia, and are a common complaint in the older age groups; one-quarter of one elderly population had some degree of sicca symptoms, affecting either the eyes or mouth. Sicca symptoms are particularly common in patients treated with anti-cholinergic agents, including many antidepressants.

## Management of Sjögren's syndrome

### Symptomatic therapy of sicca syndrome

Symptomatic therapy of sicca syndrome in SS consists of local treatment such as artificial tears and oral sprays and of systemic therapy with muscarinic agents. Several studies have demonstrated an improvement in symptoms and/or tear production. Cevimeline, a muscarinic agonist with selective high affinity towards M1 and M3 receptors, which are predominant in exocrine glands, is also effective. Ciclosporin A eye drops may be efficacious in kerato-conjuncitivitis sicca but need further evaluation.

### *Immunosuppressive therapy*

Low-dose corticosteroids are widely used in SS, although evidence from controlled studies is lacking. Hydroxychloroquine (HCQ) was found to have no beneficial effect on salivary and tear gland function compared to placebo in a 2-year double-blind crossover trial with 19 patients, which is in contrast to a retrospective open-label study by Fox (2005), who found improvement in symptoms such as sicca, arthralgia, and myalgia, but no objective tests were undertaken to confirm the improvement in these symptoms. There are no controlled studies available for azathioprine (AZA), methotrexate (MTX), and lefluonamide. Ciclosporin A orally had no effect on objective parameters to assess salivary and tear gland function.

Severe organ manifestations in SS such as myelopathy or renal involvement (interstitial nephritis) and secondary vasculitis are treated with cyclophosphamide (CYC) and corticosteroid pulses, although trial evidence is lacking. There is only one open study, including 14 patients with myelopathy in SS, which demonstrated a stabilization of walking distance and disability scores after CYC therapy. No objective parameters were measured to underline the effectiveness.

In conclusion, despite the lack of evidence SS can be treated like lupus with low-dose corticosteroids, HCQ, and immunosuppressants such as AZA, MTX, lefluonamide, and ciclosporin A for nonlife-threatening disease such as arthralgia/arthritis. CYC therapy is recommendable for organ-threatening disease, such as renal or central nervous system involvement and secondary vasculitis.

### *'Biologicals'*

So far, TNF-blocking agents have not proven to be effective in SS. Randomized double-blind controlled studies of infliximab and etanercept did not demonstrate any benefit in objective parameters testing tear and salivary gland function, in biopsy specimens and laboratory tests (ESR).

Rituximab may be a promising agent to tackle SS. Several reports have suggested a role for rituximab in SS-associated lymphoma. Furthermore, in an open-label phase II study including primary SS patients without lymphoma and patients with SS plus associated MALT lymphoma, an improvement in salivary gland function was observed as well as effective control of lymphoma.

## Summary

SS is a common autoimmune disease, which presents either alone as primary disease, or secondary to another autoimmune condition. It is characterized by diminished secretions from the salivary and lacrimal glands, which causes the hallmark symptoms of dry eyes and dry mouth. It is associated with many extraglandular features and an increased risk of development of lymphoma. Certain subtypes of the condition may be identified by the presence of particular circulating autoantibodies. There are clear diagnostic criteria, which take into account the many conditions that mimic SS. Treatment involves symptomatic and immunosuppressive therapy.

## Further reading

Akpek EK, Lindsley KB, Adyanthaya RS, *et al.* (2011). Treatment of Sjögren's Syndrome-Associated Dry Eye An Evidence-Based Review. *Ophthalmology* April 2.

Bayetto K, Logan RM (2010). Sjögren's syndrome: a review of aetiology, pathogenesis, diagnosis and management. *Aust Dent J* June;**55** Suppl 1:39–47.

Fox, RI (2005). Sjögren's syndrome. *Lancet* **366**:321–31.

Kassan SS, Moutsopoulos HM (2004). Clinical manifestations and early diagnosis of Sjögren's syndrome. *Arch Int Med* **164**:1275–84.

Amissah-Arthur MB, Gordon C (2010). Contemporary treatment of systemic lupus erythematosus: an update for clinicians. *Thera Advan Chron Dis* November;**1**:163–75.

Meijer JM, Meiners PM, Vissink A, *et al.* (2010). Effectiveness of rituximab treatment in primary Sjögren's syndrome: a randomized, double-blind, placebo-controlled trial. *Arthritis Rheum* April;**62**(4):960–8.

Ng WF, Bowman SJ (2011). Biological therapies in primary Sjögren's syndrome. *Expert Opin Biol* Ther April 4.

Ramos-Casals M, Brito-Zeron P, Font J (2007). Lessons from diseases mimicking Sjögren's syndrome. *Clin Rev Allergy Immunol* **32**:275–83.

Ramos-Casals M, Tzioufas AG, Stone JH, *et al.* (2010). Treatment of primary Sjögren syndrome: a systematic review. *JAMA* July 28;**304**(4):452–60.

Routsias JG, Tzioufas AG (2007). Sjögren's syndrome – study of autoantigens and autoantibodies. *Clin Rev Allergy Immunol* **32**:238–51.

Vitali *et al.* (2002). Classification criteria for Sjögren's syndrome: a revised version of the European criteria proposed by the American–European Consensus Group. *Ann Rheum Dis* **61**:554–8.

Voulgarelis M, Skopouli FN (2007). Clinical, immunologic and molecular factors predicting lymphoma development in Sjögren's syndrome patients. *Clin Rev Allergy Immunol* **32**:265–74.

# Anti-phospholipid syndrome

*Iona Meryon, Julia U Holle, Wolfgang L Gross, and Caroline Gordon*

## Definition and pathology

Anti-phospholipid syndrome (APS) is an autoimmune condition characterized by recurrent thrombotic events and poor obstetric outcomes in the presence of antibodies directed towards phospholipids and phospholipid-binding proteins. APS was first described in patients with systemic lupus erythematosus (SLE) and has since been recognized to occur in the context of other autoimmune conditions (see *Table 4.1*), termed secondary APS. The development of anti-phospholipid antibodies and their clinical sequelae may be independent of any underlying disease process (primary APS).

The anti-phospholipid antibodies come from a large family of autoantibodies which bind negatively charged phospholipids. Lupus anticoagulant, anti-cardiolipin and β2 glycoprotein antibodies appear to be the clinically significant antibodies. Their binding is cofactor dependent; for example, lupus anticoagulant requires prothrombin and the cofactor for anticardiolipin is β2 glycoprotein.

The precise way these autoantibodies cause thrombosis is unknown. However, four plausible mechanisms have been described:

1 Disruption of prostaglandin E2 and thromboxane production by binding endothelial structures.
2 Upregulation of platelet aggregation by binding platelet phospholipids.
3 Dysregulation of complement activation.
4 Impaired embryonic implantation and placental development due to trophoblast syncytium binding.

## Epidemiology

The prevalence of APS is unknown. Low titres of anti-cardiolipin antibodies are found in 5% of normal blood donors, and moderate to high (diagnostic levels) are found in 0.2%. In SLE they are a common finding, in up to 40% of patients. Thrombotic disorders (such as transient ischaemic attacks [TIAs], strokes, and myocardial infarctions [MI]) and complications in pregnancy are also common. It is unknown the extent to which these conditions are attributable to APS in the general population. It is likely that the disease is undiagnosed in many.

### Consensus diagnostic criteria

The Updated Sapporo APS Classification Criteria are used for the diagnosis of APS. They require a clinically significant event in the presence of a persistent laboratory abnormality. The criteria are shown in *Table 4.2*.

| Table 4.1 Rheumatic conditions associated with secondary APS |
| --- |
| SLE |
| Sjögren's syndrome |
| Dermatomyositis |
| Systemic sclerosis |
| Rheumatoid arthritis |
| Vasculitis |

## Table 4.2 The updated Sapporo Classification Criteria for anti-phospholipid syndrome

**Clinical event**
- Vascular thrombosis
- Objective evidence of clinical episode of arterial, venous, or small-vessel thrombosis in any organ or tissue

- Pregnancy event, one of:
- Three consecutive miscarriages
- Unexplained fetal death beyond 10 weeks
- Premature delivery (before 34 weeks) due to:
    Eclampsia or pre-eclampsia
    Placental insufficiency

**Laboratory abnormality**
Two positive results, 12 weeks apart
- Lupus anticoagulant
- Anti-cardiolipin IgG or IgM antibodies: moderate to high titre
- Anti-β2 glycoprotein IgG or IgM antibodies: moderate to high titre

## Table 4.3 Features suggestive of APS

Recurrent arterial and venous thromboses

Thrombosis <45 yr

Venous thromboses other than deep vein thrombosis

Arterial thrombosis in the absence of atherosclerosis

## Table 4.4 Frequency of sites for arterial thrombosis in APS

| Site of arterial thrombosis | Proportion |
| --- | --- |
| Stroke/TIA | 50% |
| Coronary thrombosis | 25% |
| Other (eye, kidney, mesentery, periphery) | 25% |

## Clinical presentation of anti-phospholipid syndrome

### Thrombosis

In APS, arterial and venous thrombosis occur in small, medium, and large vessels, producing a diverse range of clinical features (**4.1**). Venous thrombosis is the most common manifestation of APS (it occurs in over half of patients with APS), usually in the deep veins of the legs (DVT), and may be accompanied by pulmonary thromboembolism. Other sites include the renal, hepatic, axillary, ocular, and sagittal veins and the inferior vena cava. Arterial thromboses predominantly involve the brain, causing TIAs and strokes (**4.2**). These are recurrent in one-third of patients. However, they may also cause premature coronary thrombosis or infarction of intra-abdominal organs (*Tables 4.3, 4.4*).

### Pregnancy

Complications of pregnancy are a major feature of APS. The live birth rate may be as little as 10% in untreated APS; appropriate treatment increases this to about 75%. The primary mechanism by which this is thought to occur is by

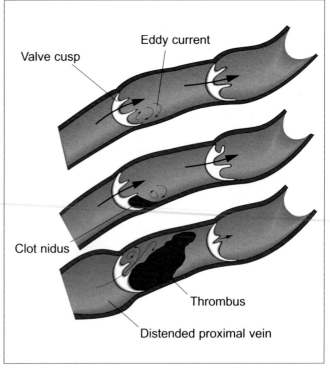

**4.1** Drawing of blood vessel showing clot formation in a vein.

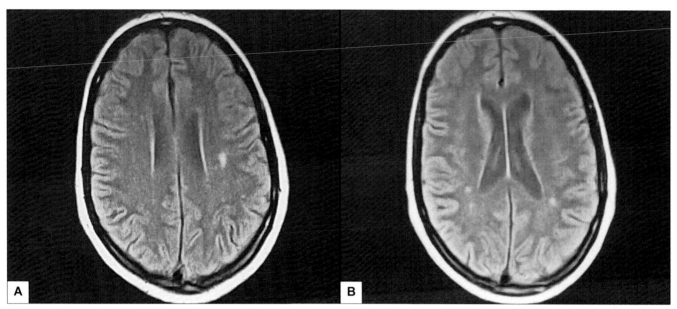

**4.2A, B**: MR brain scan of a patient with cerebrovascular accidents.

thrombosis of the placental vessels, which impairs fetal growth and causes pre-eclampsia, placental abruption, premature delivery, and miscarriages. APS affects pregnancy in three main ways: early pregnancy loss (before 10 weeks' gestation), late pregnancy loss (after 10 weeks' gestation), and premature delivery.

### Early pregnancy loss

Early pregnancy losses are common among women in the general population. It is estimated that one-quarter of pregnancies miscarry. Genetic abnormalities, such as parental chromosome and embryonic abnormalities, endocrine disorders, bacterial vaginosis, and cervical incompetence are common causes of recurrent pregnancy loss. One percent of normal women are positive for anti-phospholipid antibodies. A single early pregnancy loss is more frequently due to infection or chromosomal abnormalities, but around 10% may be attributable to APS. The likely mechanism by which early pregnancy loss occurs in APS is binding of anti-phospholipid antibodies to the trophoblast syncytium, preventing implantation. Where there is supportive laboratory evidence, a diagnosis of APS is made in someone who has had three or more unexplained, consecutive spontaneous abortions before 10 weeks' gestation, once anatomical, hormonal, and chromosomal causes for the pregnancy loss have been excluded.

### Late pregnancy loss

Late pregnancy loss may be due to congenital malformations or abnormalities of the placenta and umbilical cord. Another important cause of late pregnancy loss is cervical incompetence. APS is a significant cause of pregnancy loss after 10 weeks' gestation. The most likely mechanism is thrombosis of the placental vessels, causing placental insufficiency that results in fetal demise. Therefore, where there is no other explanation for the loss of a fetus that grossly appears normal (by direct examination or on ultrasound assessment) and particularly when there is placental infarction, APS needs to be considered as a cause of late fetal loss and appropriate investigations undertaken.

### Premature delivery

APS may also be associated with the premature delivery, defined as before 34 weeks' gestation, of a normal appearing baby though the baby may be small for dates. Apart from causing fetal demise, placental dysfunction due to APS may be associated with other obstetric complications such as pre-eclampsia, placental abruption, and intrauterine growth restriction that can lead to delivery. Although there are strict definitions of pre-eclampsia and eclampsia, there is no universal definition for placental insufficiency, and the timing of delivery is subject to the obstetrician's judgement. However, the diagnostic criteria

**Table 4.5 Consensus Criteria definitions of APS features in pregnancy (Updated Sapporo Guidelines, 2006)**

1 Three or more consecutive spontaneous abortions before 10 weeks' gestation, in the absence of an anatomical, genetic, or chromosomal cause

2 An unexplained death of a normal-appearing fetus (by ultrasound or direct examination) after 10 weeks' gestation

3 Premature delivery (before 34 weeks) of a morphologically normal fetus due to:
– Eclampsia or pre-eclampsia
– Recognized features of placental insufficiency

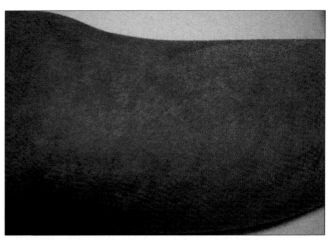

**4.3** Livedo reticularis.

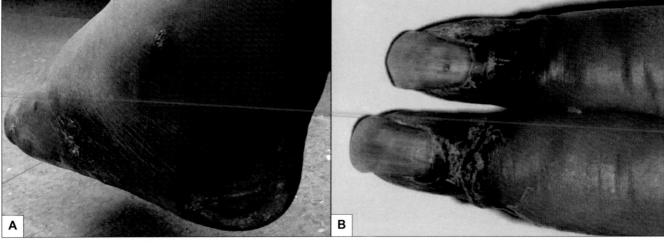

**4.4A**: Ulceration on the heel of a patient with transverse myelitis due to APS; **B**: digital gangrene in a patient with APS.

for APS provide an objective method of identifying premature deliveries that are most likely to have resulted from APS (*Tables 4.2, 4.5*).

The obstetric complications used in the APS classification criteria are common and are not specific to APS. There may be alternative causes for pregnancy loss, growth restriction due to placental insufficiency, and pre-eclampsia as these conditions may affect 10% of all pregnancies, and often lead to premature delivery in otherwise healthy women. The underlying causes in these women include smoking, alcohol abuse, and pre-existing medical conditions, such as hypertension, diabetes, and cardiac and renal disease. In the context of secondary APS, SLE disease activity may also be associated with complications in late pregnancy, including placental insufficiency.

## Skin

Cutaneous manifestations may be as the first feature of APS: livedo reticularis is the most common of these (**4.3**). It is a persistent skin change with a characteristic violaceous lacy pattern affecting the trunk, arms, and legs (*Table 4.6*). It does not reverse on rewarming and is also associated with other autoimmune conditions, cryoglobulinaemia, hyper-calcaemia, and certain infections. Other features of APS in the skin include ulceration (**4.4A**), digital gangrene (**4.4B**), purpura (see Chapter 1, **1.18**, **1.19A**, **B**), thrombophlebitis, and splinter haemorrhages (see Chapter 7, **7.33**).

### Table 4.6 Features of livedo reticularis

Persistent

Nonreversible with warming

Violaceous, red, or blue

Reticular or mottled

Regular unbroken circles or irregular broken circles

## Haematological

Thrombocytopenia is a common finding amongst patients with APS, more so when secondary to SLE. It is usually mild ($60–100 \times 10^9$ platelets/l) and rarely severe enough to cause significant bleeding. Paradoxically it is associated with an increased risk of thrombosis, and the thrombocytopenia is thought to result from platelet consumption. A low platelet count may be the presenting feature of APS, and other causes must be excluded. Anti-phospholipid antibodies are found in one-quarter of patients with immune thrombocytopenic purpura (ITP) and are associated with an increased risk of thrombosis. Therefore, patients with thrombocytopenia and persistent anti-phospholipid antibodies are termed 'anti-phospholipid antibody-associated thrombocytopenia' and warrant closer follow-up. Other haematologic features of APS include haemolytic anaemia and positive direct Coombs' test.

## Cardiac lesions

APS has several cardiac manifestations: valvular lesions, myocardial involvement, coronary artery disease, systemic and pulmonary hypertension. Valve lesions are common in APS: valvulopathy is present in almost one-half of patients with APS, and seems to be independent of any underlying SLE. Morphologically, there are two discrete abnormalities on echocardiogram: vegetations and valvular thickening, which usually causes mitral regurgitation, but is rarely severe enough to cause symptoms or warrant valve replacement. Myocardial involvement is rare. However, cases with biopsy-proven myocardial microthrombus or intracardiac thrombi would fulfil the thrombosis criterion for classification.

APS can contribute to accelerated atherosclerosis which manifests as premature ischaemic heart disease in patients without other risk factors. Coronary thrombosis fulfils the

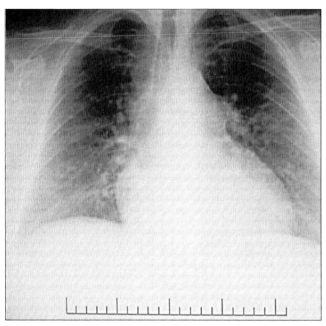

**4.5** Chest X-ray of a patient with breathlessness on exertion showing enlarged pulmonary arteries due to recurrent pulmonary emboli causing pulmonary hypertension.

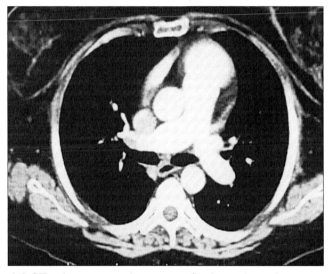

**4.6** CT pulmonary angiogram confirming enlarged pulmonary arteries in the patient in **4.5** with pulmonary hypertension secondary to recurrent pulmonary emboli.

classification criteria. Hypertension in APS may be secondary to renal artery stenosis or thrombotic microangiopathy. Recurrent pulmonary emboli can cause pulmonary hypertension (**4.5, 4.6**).

### Neurological and ophthalmic features

TIAs and strokes fulfil the classification criteria for thrombosis. However, the neurological manifestations of the condition are not limited to those used in the diagnosis. Cognitive dysfunction, seizures, chorea, and transverse myelopathy are well-recognized neurological features that occur in a small proportion of patients (*Table 4.7*). Anti-phospholipid antibodies have been used as a risk factor for dementia and cognitive impairment. In patients with cerebral involvement or transverse myelopathy, multiple sclerosis (MS)-like lesions may be seen on MR scans of the brain and spinal cord (**4.7, 4.8**). Retinal vein thrombosis may occur and it is important not to ignore manifestations of transient visual disturbance, as this can occur before permanent ischaemic damage develops (**4.9–4.11**).

**Table 4.7 Neurological features of APS**

Dementia

Cognitive impairment

Migraine

Seizures

Mood disturbance

Chorea

Myelopathy

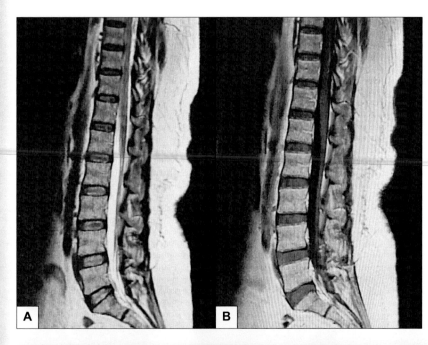

**4.7A, B**: MR scans of the spinal cord in a patient with transverse myelitis associated with APS who presented with bilateral leg weakness, numbness, and retention of urine.

**4.8A–C**: MR scans of patients with recurrent small-vessel ischaemic lesions causing severe cognitive dysfunction due to APS.

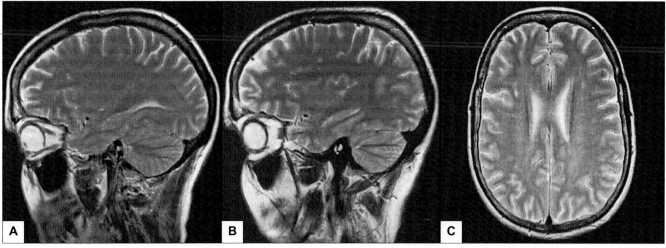

### Renal manifestations

The extent of kidney involvement is often underestimated in APS. Thrombosis of renal vasculature and intrarenal vascular lesions causes hypertension by stimulating the renin–angiotensin system. Other features of APS nephropathy are hypertension, proteinuria, haematuria, and slowly progressive renal insufficiency that may ultimately result in renal failure requiring replacement therapy (*Table 4.8*). Histologically, there are concomitant features of acute thromboses (thrombotic microangiopathy) and evidence of chronic lesions (arteriosclerosis, glomerular sclerosis, fibrous intimal hyperplasia, arteriolar occlusion, focal cortical and tubular atrophy; **4.12**). APS nephropathy may coexist with proliferative or membranous lupus nephritis in patients with SLE. Renal biopsy is the only way of establishing whether or not thrombotic microangiopathy is contributing to the clinical manifestations.

| Table 4.8 Features of APS nephropathy |
| --- |
| Low-grade proteinuria |
| Microscopic haematuria |
| Hypertension |
| Slowly progressive renal impairment |

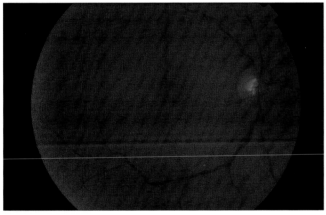

**4.9** Right fundus in a patient with a nonischaemic retinal vein thrombosis causing intermittent blurring of central vision with engorged veins and aneurysms on fundoscopy.

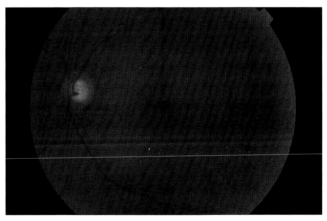

**4.10** Normal left fundus of the patient in **4.9**.

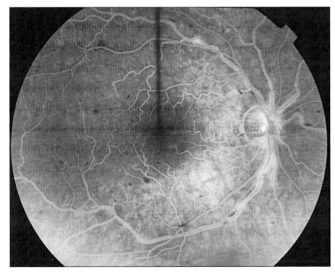

**4.11** Fluorescein angiogram of the right fundus of the patient in **4.9** highlighting dilated veins.

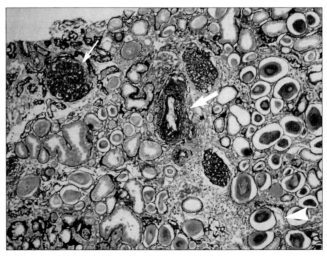

**4.12** Renal biopsy from a patient with APS showing global glomerular sclerosis (small arrow), vascular damage (large arrow), and tubular atrophy (arrowhead).

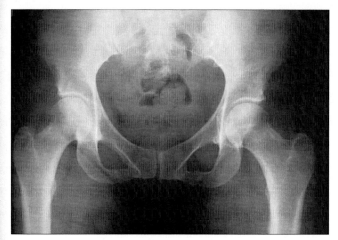

**4.13** Plain X-ray showing early aseptic necrosis of left hip.

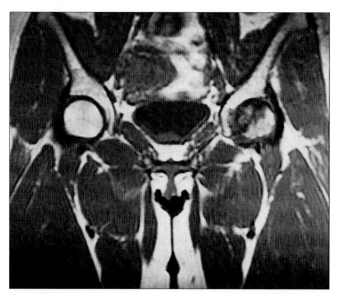

**4.14** MR scan of the left hip shown in **4.13** 6 months later, showing marked necrosis of the femoral head.

### Osteonecrosis of the hip

APS can also cause ischaemic osteonecrosis (aseptic necrosis) of the hip and has been seen in patients who have not received steroids. As plain X-ray does not show typical features early in the disease course (**4.13**), MR scan is the investigation of choice (**4.14**). In unexplained cases of aseptic osteonecrosis, APS should be considered in the differential diagnosis.

### Catastrophic APS

A small group of patients with APS develop a multiorgan disease of rapid onset (*Table 4.9*). In this severe form of disease, there is widespread deposition of microthrombi in the vascular beds of several organs, usually the lungs, central nervous system (CNS), kidneys, and mesentery. The heart, liver, and adrenal glands are less commonly involved. Patients with catastrophic APS often require organ support in intensive care facilities, and the resulting multiorgan failure gives the condition a 60% mortality rate.

Classification criteria for catastrophic APS have been devised which require all of:
- Vascular thrombosis in three or more organs and tissues.
- Development of simultaneous manifestations within 1 week.
- Evidence of small-vessel thrombosis in at least one organ or tissue.
- Laboratory evidence of anti-phospholipid antibodies.

## Differential diagnosis

APS is characterized by diverse clinical and biological features, and overlaps between rheumatology, immunology, haematology, obstetric medicine, neurology, nephrology, and molecular biology. The criteria require a clinical event in the context of persistent laboratory evidence of anti-phospholipid antibodies. However, the diagnostic autoantibodies are common in the normal population, as are complications of pregnancy and thrombotic events. There are many causes of obstetric complications, thrombotic events, and false-positive laboratory evidence. The other causes of obstetric complications have already been discussed.

### Thrombosis

There are many conditions predisposing to thrombus formation (*Table 4.10*). These need to be excluded before attributing an episode of thrombosis to APS. The oral contraceptive is responsible for the majority of cases in young women. Hormone replacement therapy is associated with a 2–4-fold risk. Underlying malignancy accounts for up to one-fifth of cases of venous thrombosis. Anti-coagulant factor deficiency is less common and affects less than 1% of the population. In many prothrombotic states (such as protein C, S, and antithrombin III deficiency), thrombosis occurs only in the venous system, and cannot account for arterial thrombosis.

**Table 4.9 Manifestations of catastrophic APS**

| Site involved | Features |
|---|---|
| Lungs | Respiratory failure<br>ARDS |
| CNS | Stroke<br>TIA |
| Renal | Acute renal failure<br>Malignant hypertension |
| Gastrointestinal tract | Mesenteric ischaemia |
| Heart | MI, cardiac arrest |
| Peripheries | Cutaneous infarction |
| Adrenal | Acute adrenal insufficiency |
| Liver | Acute ischaemic hepatitis |

**Table 4.10 Some other prothrombotic conditions**

Oral contraceptive pill and hormone replacement therapy

Malignancy

Factor V Leiden mutation

Protein C and S deficiency

**Table 4.11 Nonautoimmune causes of anti-phospholipid antibody production**

| Infections | Drugs |
|---|---|
| Lyme disease | Calcium channel blockers |
| Leptospirosis | Phenytoin |
| Syphilis | Isoniazid |
| Epstein–Barr | |
| HIV | |
| Pinta | |

### Positive anti-phospholipid antibodies

Anti-phospholipid antibodies are common findings and, alone, do not represent anti-phospholipid syndrome. Elevated antibody levels are not always clinically significant; often they are low titre and transient following infection. Moderate to high titre of IgG and IgM anti-cardiolipin antibodies is associated with a risk of pulmonary embolism eight times that of the population with negative tests. Of the three autoantibodies, lupus anticoagulant confers the highest risk of thrombotic complications.

There is diagnostic uncertainty about the significance of anti-phospholipid antibodies in the elderly, as thrombotic events and positive tests both occur at greater frequency. It may be unclear whether the event is attributable to known traditional risk factors (such as smoking) or APS. Anti-phospholipid antibodies may occur in conditions such as lymphoproliferative disease, end-stage renal disease, and infections, and may be caused by certain drugs (*Table 4.11*) with an uncertain risk of causing thrombosis. Where infection triggers autoantibody production, they are usually transient and IgM predominant. Individuals with drug-induced anti-phospholipid antibodies which persist after withdrawal of the drug are at an increased risk of thrombosis.

## Management of anti-phospholipid syndrome

### Therapy for nonpregnant patients

There is no evidence for a specific antithrombotic prophylactic therapy for patients with anti-phospholipid antibodies who have not suffered from a thrombotic event. Secondary prophylaxis after a thrombotic event in APS demands anticoagulation. Medication and intensity of anticoagulation are dependent on the localization of thrombosis (*Table 4.12*). For secondary prophylaxis of DVT, warfarin with a target international normalized ratio (INR) of 2–3 is sufficient to reduce the risk of recurring thrombosis by about 85%. A retrospective trial addressed the question of whether aspirin or low-intensity warfarin may be used as secondary prophylaxis in DVT due to APS. It was found that aspirin and low-intensity warfarin were probably less efficient compared to moderate or high-intensity anticoagulation. In summary, moderate anti-coagulation with a target INR of 2–3 is the treatment of choice for the prevention of recurring DVT.

Arterial thrombosis may occur in a variety of organs. Although one study suggested that secondary prophylaxis with low- to moderate-intensity anticoagulation with warfarin is as efficient as aspirin 325 mg/day for preventing

**Table 4.12 Guide to treatment of APS in nonpregnant patients with oral anticoagulation, e.g. warfarin**

| Event | Target INR on anticoagulation |
|---|---|
| First venous thrombosis or pulmonary embolus | 2–3 |
| Recurrent venous thrombosis or pulmonary emboli off anticoagulation | 2–3 |
| Recurrent venous thrombosis or pulmonary embolus on anticoagulation with INR 2–3 | 3–4 |
| Arterial thrombosis (not associated with atherosclerosis) | 3–4 |

**Table 4.13 Guide to treatment of APS in pregnant patients**

| Event | Intervention |
|---|---|
| No previous thrombosis, cardiac valve disease or fetal loss | None |
| One or two fetal losses at <10 weeks' gestation with no other thrombotic events | Low-dose aspirin (e.g. 75 mg/day) |
| Recurrent fetal losses (three or more) attributable to APS at <10 weeks' gestation with no other thrombotic events | Low-dose aspirin (e.g. 75 mg/day) and/or prophylactic subcutaneous low-molecular-weight heparin |
| Fetal loss at >10 weeks' gestation attributable to APS | Low-dose aspirin (e.g. 75 mg/day) and prophylactic subcutaneous low-molecular-weight heparin |
| Recurrent fetal losses at >10 weeks' gestation attributable to APS despite low-dose aspirin and subcutaneous heparin at prophylactic dose | Consider low-dose aspirin (e.g. 75 mg/day) and therapeutic subcutaneous low-molecular-weight heparin |
| Previous venous thrombosis outside of pregnancy and not on regular anticoagulation before pregnancy | Low-dose aspirin (e.g. 75 mg/day) and prophylactic subcutaneous low-molecular-weight heparin |
| Previous venous or arterial thrombosis or cardiac valve disease outside of pregnancy treated with routine oral anticoagulation before pregnancy | Low-dose aspirin (e.g. 75 mg/day) and therapeutic subcutaneous low-molecular-weight heparin |

recurrent cerebral events, moderate- or high-intensity anticoagulation is usually recommended, particularly for patients with cardiac and gastrointestinal ischaemic events, young patients with stroke, and those with renal artery stenosis. Management of renal thrombotic micro-angiopathy requires investigation, as this is becoming an increasingly recognized cause of renal failure, but there is little evidence to support the use of warfarin. Hydroxy-chloroquine may have some effect in reducing thrombotic events and antibody titre in APS. Rituximab has been used to treat refractory APS, according to a few case reports. Duration of anticoagulation is usually recommended to be lifelong in the absence of a contraindication but there is no evidence from trials for the duration of therapy.

### Therapy for pregnant patients

Patients who have experienced recurrent pregnancy losses (at least three) in the first 10 weeks of pregnancy attributed to APS usually receive low-dose aspirin (e.g. 75 mg/day). For patients with recurrent early losses despite aspirin and for those with losses after week 10 of pregnancy due to APS, low-dose aspirin in combination with subcutaneous heparin (preferably low-molecular-weight heparin) in prophylactic dose is usually used (*Table 4.13*). For patients with a history of any thrombotic event associated with APS (venous or arterial), subcutaneous heparin (preferably low-molecular-weight heparin) in therapeutic dose is usually used. Heparin should not be stopped until 6 weeks postpartum due to the increased risk of thrombosis in the early postpartum period, though it will need to be discontinued temporarily at the time of delivery. Whether pregnant women who are anti-phospholipid antibody-positive but who do not have a history of thrombotic events or fetal losses need prophylactic therapy is not known, but low-dose aspirin is often prescribed. The use of intravenous immunoglobulin (IVIG) in pregnant women has not proven effective in preventing recurrent pregnancy loss.

## Summary

APS is an immune disorder of coagulation, characterized by thrombosis, adverse pregnancy outcomes, and production of autoantibodies to anti-phospholipids. It occurs both as an isolated condition and secondary to autoimmune disease, such as SLE. Diagnosis requires a clinical event of thrombosis or certain complications of pregnancy in the context of persistent laboratory evidence of anti-phospholipid antibodies. Other features have also been described, such as thrombocytopenia, livedo reticularis, and nephropathy. Treatment has been summarized in *Tables 4.12* and *4.13*.

## Further reading

Asherson RA, Cervera R, de Groot PG, *et al.* (2003). Catastrophic antiphospholipid syndrome: international consensus statement on classification criteria and treatment guideline. *Lupus* **12**:530–4.

Black A (2006). Antiphospholipid syndrome: an overview. *Clin Lab Sci* **19**(3):144.

Cohen H, Machin SJ (2010). Antithrombotic treatment failures in antiphospholipid syndrome: the new anticoagulants? *Lupus* April;**19**(4):486–91.

Hanly JG (2003). Antiphospholipid syndrome: an overview. *CMAJ* **168**(13):1675–82.

Miyakis S, Lockshin MD, Atsumi T, Branch DW, *et al.* (2006). International consensus statement on an update of the classification criteria for definite antiphospholipid syndrome (APS). *J Thromb Haemost* **4**:295–306.

Ruiz-Irastorza G, Crowther M, Branch W, Khamashta MA (2010). Antiphospholipid syndrome. *Lancet* October 30;**376**(9751):1498–509.

Scoble T, Wijetilleka S, Khamashta MA (2010). Management of refractory anti-phospholipid syndrome. *Autoimmun Rev* May 1.

Tuthill JI, Khamashta MA (2009). Management of antiphospholipid syndrome. *J Autoimmun* **33**(2):92–8.

Vashisht A, Regan L (2005). Antiphospholipid syndrome in pregnancy – an update. *J R Coll Phys Edin* **35**:337–9.

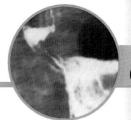
# Idiopathic inflammatory myopathies

*Iona Meryon, Julia U Holle, Wolfgang L Gross, and Caroline Gordon*

## Definition and classification

The idiopathic inflammatory myopathies (IIMs) are a spectrum of muscle diseases that are classified further by their clinical and histological features. There are three typical features of all the IIMs: symmetrical proximal muscle weakness, reduced muscle endurance, and nonsuppurative skeletal muscle inflammation (**5.1**).

Polymyositis (PM) and dermatomyositis (DM) can occur alone or in association with connective tissue diseases (CTDs) or malignancy. Systemic sclerosis (SSc) is the most common CTD associated with an inflammatory myopathy, but there are also associations with systemic lupus erythematosus (SLE), rheumatoid arthritis, Sjögren's syndrome (SS), and mixed CTD. DM may occur in children and later in life may occur with malignancy. When myositis is associated with other types of systemic autoimmune disease (such as Crohn's, hypothyroidism, or coeliac disease) it usually manifests as PM. Skin involvement occurs infrequently. Infections and drugs can also cause muscle inflammation; these causes are not discussed here.

PM and DM account for the majority of cases of IIM. Inclusion body myositis (IBM) has been described more recently, and other rare types include focal nodular myositis, eosinophilic myositis, and myositis ossificans (*Table 5.1*). DM is distinguished clinically from PM by the presence of characteristic skin features: the heliotrope rash and Gottron's papules.

A system of classification was described in 1975 (Bohan and Peter), and a few revisions have been made since, shown in sections VI and VII of *Table 5.1*.

The main role of this classification system is to predict the course of the disease and the response to treatment. There is significant clinical overlap between these conditions which themselves can often present atypically, and this makes further classification of IIM difficult. Since Bohan and Peter's original classification system, another important differential has been explored: inclusion body myositis was described upon more detailed histological study of muscle biopsies from older patients who clinically fulfilled the criteria for PM but did not respond to treatment. Muscle biopsy identifies these patients and is important for defining prognosis and planning treatment. There are several other rare types of idiopathic myositis which must also be considered, including focal nodular myositis, eosinophilic myositis, and myositis ossificans. These are discussed later.

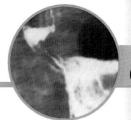

**5.1** Characteristic features of inflammatory myopathies.

**Table 5.1 Revised classification of inflammatory myopathies (after Bohan & Peter, 1975)**

| | | |
|---|---|---|
| *Original classification system* | I | Primary idiopathic polymyositis |
| | II | Primary idiopathic dermatomyositis |
| | III | Polymyositis/dermatomyositis associated with malignancy |
| | IV | Juvenile polymyositis/dermatomyositis |
| | V | Overlap syndrome of polymyositis/dermatomyositis with another connective tissue disease |
| *Later additions to classification system* | VI | Inclusion body myositis |
| | VII | Rare forms of myositis include:<br>• Focal nodular myositis<br>• Eosinophilic myositis<br>• Myositis ossificans |

## Epidemiology

Inflammatory myopathy is an uncommon disease, with an estimated prevalence of 1 in 100,000. However, it is the most common (and often treatable) cause of acquired skeletal muscle weakness and can be associated with other autoimmune and CTDs. DM is distinguishable by the additional feature of characteristic skin lesions.

There is a bimodal age distribution for all cases of IIM, with an initial peak in adolescence and another at 40–60 years (**5.2**). The majority of cases of PM and DM occur in 50–60-year-olds. When inflammatory myositis presents in the older age group, there is a signficant risk that it is associated with an underlying malignancy. There is a female to male ratio of 2:1 (which rises to a ratio of 5:1 during childbearing years) and a marked ethnic variation in the distribution of inflammatory myopathy. It is most common in African-Americans, and lowest rates are observed in those of Japanese origin (*Table 5.2*). DM increases relative to PM

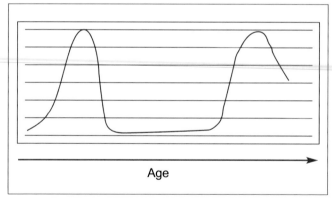

**5.2** Bimodal age distribution of IIMs with peaks in adolescence and age 40–60 years.

**Table 5.2 Typical epidemiological features of polymyositis, dermatomyositis, and inclusion body myositis**

| | *Polymyositis* | *Dermatomyositis* | *Inclusion body myositis* |
|---|---|---|---|
| Age | Over 20 | Children and adults | Over 50 |
| Sex | Women | Women | Men |
| Ethnicity | African-American | African-American | Caucasian |

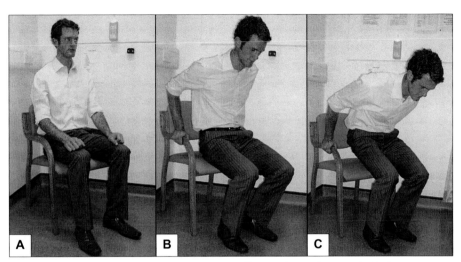

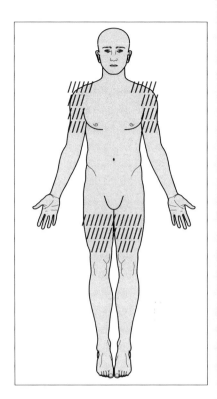

**5.4A–C**: Series of photographs showing difficulty rising from a chair due to proximal muscle weakness.

**5.3** Illustration of proximal body areas (in red) where muscles become weak in inflammatory myopathies.

at lower latitudes and there is geographical variation the prevalence of myositis-associated antibodies.

In some cases the disease onset is rapid and muscle swelling and overlying skin oedema may be observed early in the course of the disease. In such cases, there may also be myoglobinuria. Rarely, there may be a gradual onset of symptoms over several years. In such cases, it can be difficult to distinguish these from hereditary and degenerative causes of muscle weakness, such as muscular dystrophy. Although the cause of IIM is unknown, certain triggers have been observed. Patients often associate the onset of symptoms with a minor infection, such as a viral respiratory infection, and describe a prodromal phase of constitutional upset before the myopathy is apparent. A family history of idiopathic myositis is rare and hereditary muscle disease, such as Duchenne's muscular dystrophy, should be excluded first. However, there are reports of familial cases of IBM, and certain autoimmune diseases which are associated with myositis show familial patterns.

## Clinical presentation of idiopathic inflammatory myopathy

### Musculoskeletal and dermatological features
Inflammatory myositis is a multisystem disease with vague nonspecific symptoms that develop gradually: myalgia and

fatigue usually precede muscle weakness, and can be associated with systemic complaints, such as fatigue, weight loss, and anorexia. These may be the only features if patients present with early disease. Fever is more common in those patients who have anti-Jo-1 autoantibodies. The hallmark of IIM is proximal symmetrical muscle weakness. The muscle weakness principally affects the muscles of the shoulder and hip girdles (**5.3**, *Table 5.3*). Patients describe difficulty rising from a chair (**5.4A–C**), climbing stairs, and

**Table 5.3 Functional impairment associated with muscle weakness in inflammatory myopathies**

| Major muscle groups affected | Functional impairment |
| --- | --- |
| Pelvic girdle | Rising from chair Getting out of cars |
| Limb girdles | Lifting Climbing stairs, squatting |
| Shoulder girdle | Combing hair |
| Neck flexors | Holding head up |

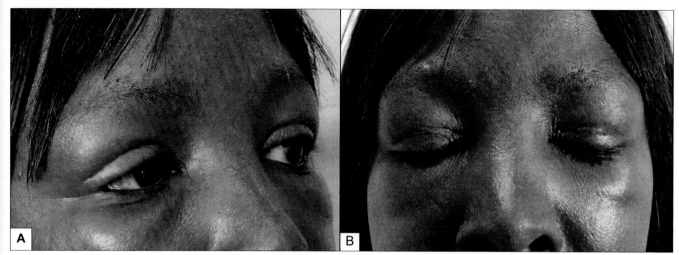

**5.5A, B**: Heliotrope rash affecting the upper eyelids and periorbital skin.

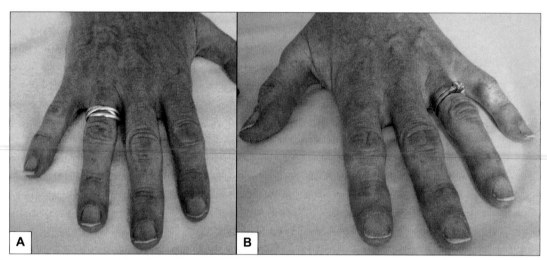

**5.6A, B**: Gottron's papules overlying the metacarpophalangeal and proximal interphalangeal joints of both hands.

brushing hair (see *Table 5.3*) and may complain of muscle tenderness. If the weakness is very mild, the only physical sign may be difficulty maintaining elevation of an arm or leg, particularly against resistance. However, due to the insidious onset of symptoms, patients usually have developed abnormal physical signs by the time they present. The myopathy can involve the bulbar muscles, impairing speech production and coordination of swallowing. The respiratory muscles may also become involved. The disease is said 'never' to affect the ocular muscles. The disease can also cause an arthralgia and early morning stiffness but these are not usually prominent features.

When PM is associated with characteristic skin lesions, it is defined as DM. There are two classical types of skin rash: the heliotrope rash and Gottrons's papules. The heliotrope rash is a dusky violaceous erythema which affects the upper eyelid margin and periorbital skin (**5.5A, B**). Gottron's papules are symmetrical lacy pink violaceous papules and plaques which lie over bony prominences, such as the metacarpophalangeal joints (**5.6A, B**) and the knees. They can be covered with a scale and have telangiectasia within the lesion.

There are many other cutaneous manifestations associated with DM (**5.7**). There are two rashes that appear in a photodistribution, but are not always due to ultraviolet light exposure: the 'shawl sign' covers the posterior aspects of the neck and shoulders, and the 'V-sign' affects the anterior surfaces of the neck and shoulders. The hand is a common site for skin changes, which include dystrophic cuticles and distinctive nailfold changes, such as periungal

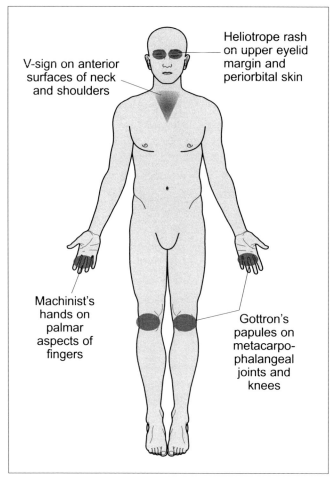

V-sign on anterior surfaces of neck and shoulders

Heliotrope rash on upper eyelid margin and periorbital skin

Machinist's hands on palmar aspects of fingers

Gottron's papules on metacarpo-phalangeal joints and knees

**5.7** Diagram illustrating the location of the different rashes that can occur in DM.

telangiectasia. 'Machinist's hands' describes darkened horizontal lines across the palmar aspects of the fingers. This feature is associated with an increased risk of interstitial lung disease.

### Physical signs on examination

The physical signs of IIM are variable in this multisystem disease. The signs may reflect the underlying disease process, the effects of treatment, and/or complications (*Table 5.4*). Documentation of muscle strength is important for assessing progression of disease activity and response to treatment. The Medical Research Council (MRC) scale for grading muscle strength in peripheral muscles is most frequently used (*Table 5.5*). There is also ongoing work to validate objective methods of measuring muscle strength by mechanical means. The disease process can directly affect the respiratory muscles: 5% of patients have respiratory muscle weakness which may require temporary ventilatory support. Weakness of the pharyngeal and oesophageal muscles may also result in aspiration pneumonia.

---

**Table 5.4 Summary of examination findings in patients with inflammatory myopathy**

***Motor function***

Reduced power – proximal, symmetrical distribution (grade via MRC scale or mechanical testing)

Tenderness over muscles

***Neurology***

Normal sensation and tone

Reflexes intact (unless late atrophic disease)

***Skin***

Heliotrope rash

Gottron's papules

Shawl sign, V sign photosensitivity

Nailfold changes

Machinist's hands

***Extramuscular***

Crackles on auscultation of chest

Arrhythmias

Dysphonia

---

**Table 5.5 Medical Research Council system for objective semiquantitative grading of muscle strength**

5 Normal power on resistance

4 Decreased power, but muscle contraction possible against resistance

3 Muscle contraction only against gravity

2 Muscle contraction only possible when gravity eliminated

1 Muscle contraction, but no motion

0 No muscle contraction

### Nonmusculoskeletal features

IIM is a multisystem disease that affects many organs and tissues other than the musculoskeletal system and skin (**5.8**).

### Pulmonary complications

Up to one-half of patients with IIM have respiratory complications. The aetiology of such complications is usually due to one or a combination of: interstitial lung disease (ILD), intrinsic respiratory muscle weakness, or iatrogenic causes.

ILD complicates around 30% of cases of PM and DM (**5.9, 5.10**). The pattern of the lung involvement mimics that of other CTDs – interstitial fibrosis mainly affecting the lung bases, and chest radiography shows a reticulonodular pattern in the bases. However, the severity of lung disease is not related to disease activity and can range from radiological findings in an asymptomatic patient to a condition similar to end-stage pulmonary fibrosis. It is more common if antisynthetase (Jo-1) positive and in some connective tissue overlap syndromes. High-resolution CT (HRCT) imaging detects early stages of lung involvement better than plain chest X-ray and has a role in screening for respiratory complications.

Interstitial lung fibrosis is associated with a restrictive pattern on pulmonary function testing and exercise-related hypoxaemia. Note that both ILD and respiratory muscle weakness show a restrictive pattern on lung function testing. These conditions are distinguished by assessing the transfer factor using carbon monoxide.

Finally, there are two important iatrogenic causes of respiratory involvement:

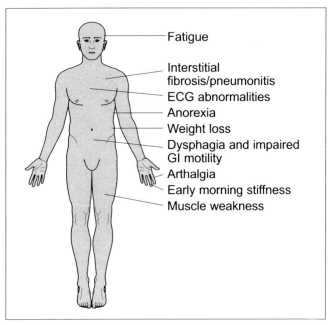

5.8 Diagram summarizing the nonskeletal features of IIM.

1 Opportunistic infections (such as *Pneumocystis carinii* pneumonia) can occur secondary to immunosuppressive agents.
2 Drug toxicity – methotrexate (MTX) and less commonly azathiaprine (AZA) can cause a pneumonitis.

### Cardiac complications

The heart is the most common nonskeletal site of involvement in IIM. Up to three-quarters of patients have some degree of cardiac involvement and the majority is asymptomatic. However, the cardiovascular risk is four

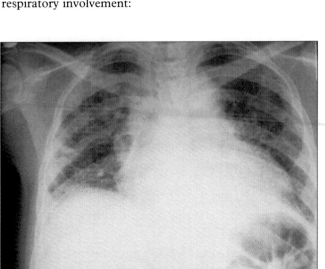

5.9 Chest X-ray of the lungs in a patient with lung fibrosis associated with inflammatory myositis.

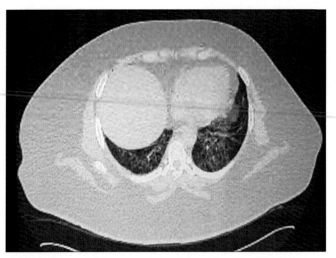

5.10 High-resolution CT scan of the lungs in a patient with lung fibrosis associated with inflammatory myositis.

times that of the normal population and cardiovascular complications are the most common cause of death of patients with myositis. There are two mechanisms by which this occurs: direct involvement of the myocardium and inflammatory acceleration of atherosclerosis.

Cardiac failure is the most common cardiovascular complication to manifest clinically and usually occurs with active muscle disease. There is a higher rate of left ventricular diastolic dysfunction compared to the general population. Small pericardial effusions are common, and cardiomyopathy has also been described. Electrocardiogram (ECG) abnormalities are found in up to 70% of patients. Although arrhythmias may be a presenting feature, the majority of ECG changes are minor nonspecific ST segment or T wave changes. Further cardiac conduction abnormalities requiring intervention (such as heart block) are rare.

### Gastrointestinal complications

The gastrointestinal (GI) complications of IIMs are generally associated with smooth muscle involvement, and the onset is usually related to active skeletal muscle disease and responds to systemic treatment. In overlap conditions, the underlying CTD such as SSc may also cause bowel involvement. When the oesophagus is involved, dysphagia and regurgitation are common features. Aspiration of gastric contents is associated with significant complications. Symptoms of gastro-oesophageal reflux occur if the gastro-oesophageal sphincter is involved and there may be some degree of dysmotility with slow clearing of the oesophagus (**5.11**). Delayed gastric emptying may occur as well. In juvenile DM, GI vasculitis causes mucosal ulceration, which presents with bleeding or perforation.

## Diagnosis

The diagnosis of inflammatory myositis depends on clinical features, laboratory and histological findings, and electromyography (EMG) studies, as shown in *Table 5.6*. The diagnosis of inflammatory myositis requires several features and diagnosis cannot be made on an individual finding. Muscle enzymes, EMG studies, and histological features are essential diagnostic investigations, and other causes of muscle disease must also be excluded.

There is an emerging role for using autoantibodies and MR studies in diagnosis. Targoff *et al.* (1997) revised Bohan and Peter's (1975) diagnostic criteria by adding myositis-specific antibodies to their five features. Their revisions also included radiological investigation in the diagnostic system,

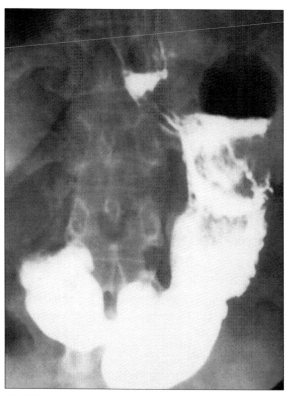

**5.11** Barium swallow in a patient with mild dysmotility and slow clearing of the oesophagus.

allowing consistent MR images to substitute for either weakness or elevated serum enzymes in the diagnosis. They proposed that the diagnosis be subdivided into:
- Definite – any four criteria.
- Probable – any three criteria.
- Possible – any two criteria.

### Variants of disease

IIM covers a spectrum of disease. Although the majority of cases follow the typical course, some variants have also been described.

### Amyopathic dermatomyositis ('dermatomyositis sine myositis')

This has been described in patients with typical cutaneous DM who develop no clinical myositis for at least 2 years without immunosuppression. However, the risks of malignancy and systemic complications such as ILD are comparable to those of dermatomyositis.

### Juvenile disease

In children, the typical skin changes of DM usually precede muscle involvement. It is associated with more systemic

**Table 5.6 Diagnostic criteria for inflammatory myositis developed by Bohan and Peter (1975)**

| *Features of muscle involvement (polymyositis)* | Weakness | Symmetrical proximal weakness, mainly affecting the limb girdles |
| --- | --- | --- |
| | Muscle enzymes | Raised  CK<br>Aldolase<br>SGOT<br>SGPT<br>LDH |
| | Histology | Fibre necrosis and regeneration, inflammatory infiltrate |
| | EMG | Triad of<br>i Fibrillations<br>ii High-frequency discharges<br>iii Short small polyphasic motor units |
| *Additional features of skin involvement (dermatomyositis)* | Dermatological features | Heliotrope rash around eyelids<br>Gottron's papules<br>Machinist's hands |

complications than the adult form of the disease, which include systemic calcification, lipodystrophy, and vasculitis. However, if the disease is limited to muscle involvement, it follows a similar course to adult polymyositis.

### Focal nodular myositis

PM may present in a focal nodular form, with painful tender nodules in the muscle which develop over a couple of weeks. Biopsy is necessary to differentiate the nodules from skeletal muscle tumours; the histological features of the nodules are identical to PM. Focal nodular myositis can resolve spontaneously or may progress to diffuse disease.

### Eosinophilic myositis

Histologically, an eosinophilic infiltrate differentiates eosinophilic myositis from classical PM. This condition presents in a similar way to PM, and may be a manifestation of a systemic hypereosinophilic syndrome. It responds well to steroids and may be a focal, relapsing, or progressive condition.

### Myositis ossificans

There are two forms of myositis ossificans. Localized disease usually results from trauma and causes calcification within the muscle. However, widespread disease is an autosomal dominant condition, and is often associated with other congenital abnormalities. Tender muscle swelling starts in childhood, and later calcifies.

## Course of disease

Typically, patients describe an insidious onset of symptoms over 3–6 months with no definite trigger. However, the presenting features can also be episodic or persistent and sudden rhabdomyolysis has been described. Strength may be unimpaired initially, with only subclinical inflammatory changes. This progression of disease is generally slower in PM than DM. When the myositis is associated with malignancy, immunosuppression is less effective and there is a poor prognosis.

### Association with malignancy

There is a significant association between idiopathic myositis and malignancy, which appears to be more closely linked to DM than PM. It may present before, during, or after the diagnosis of DM, and the muscle involvement often shows paraneoplastic features, whereby the activity of the myositis corresponds to the treatment or recurrence of the cancer. The mechanism of this association is unknown. The most common tumours associated with DM are those that are common in the population, such as lung, breast, bowel, and lymphomas (*Table 5.7*). However, ovarian cancer is over-represented in women, and the risk of such may be up to 20 times that of the general population.

The role of screening for occult malignancy and ongoing surveillance is controversial. Extensive blind radiological investigation (such as whole-body CT) for occult malignancy rarely benefits the patient. After the age of 50 years, patients are thoroughly screened for occult malignancy and investigation is tailored to the patient's age, sex, and risk factors (*Table 5.8*). Malignancy must also be excluded in a younger patient presenting with suspicious symptoms. Screening should take place at the time of diagnosis. A thorough history and examination should be performed, including digital rectal examination and urinalysis. Selected investigations (such as chest radiography, faecal occult blood test) are performed along with other risk stratified screening investigations (*Table 5.8*).

The risk of malignancy is greatest during the first year, but remains higher than the general population for 5 years. Evaluation of cancer risk and appropriate investigation are repeated annually during this time. Malignancy should be suspected if there is a poor response to immunosuppressive therapy.

### Overlap syndromes

Muscle weakness is a common problem in patients with CTD. It can result from underlying disease processes and cytokine production, or be secondary to immuno-suppressive treatment (such as steroid usage). A myositis clinically indistinguishable from PM can present in certain CTDs (*Table 5.9*). In these patients, muscle biopsy is an important investigation. Although histological features are often identical to those seen in PM, additional features related to the underlying CTD may also be seen.

## Differential diagnosis

IIM is relatively rare and there are numerous conditions that have similar clinical features. There are many causes of muscle weakness that occur commonly (*Table 5.10*). Polymyalgia rheumatica presents with stiffness and pain in the distribution of the shoulder and pelvic girdles, and a raised acute phase response. However, although pain may limit movement in the proximal muscle groups, muscle strength should not be impaired. Muscular dystrophies also present with a proximal symmetrical muscle weakness. They usually have a family history and present early in life. Limb-girdle muscular dystrophy causes proximal muscle wasting in the fourth decade of life and is therefore easily confused with PM.

**Table 5.7 Common tumours associated with inflammatory myositis**

| | |
|---|---|
| Ovarian | Gastrointestinal |
| Lung | Non-Hodgkin's lymphoma |
| Breast | |

**Table 5.8 Risk factors for malignancy in patients with inflammatory myositis and relevant screening investigations**

| *Risk factors* | *Appropriate investigations* |
|---|---|
| Female | CA-125 |
| | Pelvic ultrasound |
| | Mammogram |
| Family history bowel cancer | Colonoscopy |
| Change in bowel habit | Faecal occult blood positive |
| Asian ethnicity | Full ENT assessment for nasopharyngeal cancer |
| Smoker | Chest X-ray |

**Table 5.9 Other connective tissue diseases that may be associated with inflammatory myopathy**

Mixed connective tissue disease

SLE

Scleroderma

Rheumatoid arthritis

Sjögren's syndrome

Polymyalgia rheumatica, giant cell arteritis

Vasculitis

**Table 5.10 Differential diagnosis for patients presenting with muscle pain and/or weakness**

*Polymyalgia rheumatica*

*Muscular dystrophies*
Duchenne's, Becker's, fascioscapulohumeral
dystrophy, limb-girdle dystrophy

*Neurological disease*
Denervating disease, disorders of the neuromuscular
junction, peripheral neuropathies

*Paraneoplastic phenomena*

*Infections*
HIV, EBV, CMV, *Mycobacterium*, *Toxoplasma*

*Metabolic*
Primary (storage diseases and mitochondrial disorders)
Secondary (thyroid, parathyroid)

*Rhabdomyolysis*

*Fibromyalgia*

**Table 5.11 Causes of raised creatine kinase**

| | |
|---|---|
| Muscle disease | Metabolic disorder |
| Muscle trauma | CNS disease |
| Heavy unaccustomed exercise | Malignancy |
| | Normal variant |
| Drugs | |

Neurological conditions cause muscle weakness and can be differentiated by the asymmetrical distribution and distal involvement of muscle groups, and additional disruption to sensory or cranial nerves and reflexes. Fibromyalgia presents with chronic fatigue and generalized muscle pain and tenderness localized to classical points. Patients usually complain of sleep disturbance and have no evidence of any weakness or inflammatory features unless there is a coexisting CTD.

## Investigations

The most important tests in the investigation of suspected myositis are measurements of serum muscle enzymes, electrophysiological tests of the muscle (EMG), and histology. Autoantibodies are also used to support the diagnosis and further subclassify the myositis.

### Enzymes

Active muscle damage causes release of enzymes derived from skeletal muscle – these include creatine kinase (CK), aldolase, aspartate transaminase (AST), alanine transferase (ALT) and lactate dehydrogenase (LDH). Many conditions cause elevated serum levels of muscle enzymes, and must be interpreted in the clinical context. Important differentials include muscle trauma (such as intramuscular injections and strenuous exercise), drug-induced muscle damage (e.g. statins), and endocrine and neurological diseases (see *Table 5.11*).

Myositis is usually associated with an elevated serum CK level, usually 10 to 100 times the normal level. CK is the most sensitive measure of persistent myopathy, and is used for diagnosis and to monitor disease activity and response to treatment. These levels correlate with disease activity over time; however, they may precede clinical features by over 1 month and falling CK levels generally predates restoration of muscle strength. Although CK levels may be normal in active myositis (particularly so in DM), 95% of myositis patients have a raised CK at some point in the course of their disease. In late-stage disease, the CK rise associated with active myositis is less dramatic due to muscle atrophy. CK isoenzymes have been used to identify whether the enzymes originate from skeletal muscle or cardiac. However, over one-half of PM patients have a raised CK-MB without cardiac involvement – troponin assays have emerged as a useful investigation to differentiate cardiac involvement.

Adolase may be elevated but does not correlate well with disease activity. LDH, AST, and ALT may correlate with active myositis but are less sensitive than CK. Carbonic anhydrase III is found exclusively in skeletal muscle and also rises in myositis.

Although not an enzyme, myoglobin is an oxygen-binding haeme protein that is specific to skeletal muscle, and its role in predicting exacerbations has been described. In active myositis, serum myoglobin levels may be raised without a corresponding elevated CK level, even when myoglobin is undetectable in the urine.

**Table 5.12 Autoantibodies that can be associated with inflammatory myositis**

| Class | Definition | Autoantibody examples |
|---|---|---|
| Myositis-specific autoantibodies (MSAs) | Specific to polymyositis/dermatomyositis | Antisynthetases (e.g. anti-Jo-1)<br>Antisignal recognition peptide<br>Anti-Mi-2 |
| Myositis-associated autoantibodies (MAAs) | Specific to connective tissue diseases with a myositis overlap | Anti-PM-Scl (scleroderma)<br>Anti-SnRNPs (overlap CTD)<br>Anti Ro/La (SLE, Sjögren's)<br>Anti-Ku (scleroderma, SLE) |

## Autoantibodies

As with many CTDs, PM and DM are typified by circulating autoantibodies, which are found in over 90% of patients. There are many autoantibodies associated with inflammatory myopathy, which can be subclassed either as specific to IIM (MSA), or associated with myositis (MAA). Currently, tests for the majority of these autoantibodies are not routinely available (see *Table 5.12*).

Rheumatoid factor and anti-nuclear antibody (ANA) are the most common autoantibodies, present in one-half of cases. ANA is more commonly associated with overlapping CTDs, and these are usually accompanied by other MAAs.

### Myositis-specific autoantibodies

One-quarter of patients have MSA. The immune globulins target nuclear and cytoplasmic antigens, mainly via antisynthetase, antisignal recognition peptide, and anti-Mi-2 antibodies.

Patients generally produce only one form of MSA. The antibody produced identifies a homogeneous group of patients in whom certain features of the disease predominate (*Table 5.13*).

Anti-Jo-1 antibody was the first MSA in clinical use. It is highly specific for PM, and less commonly for DM. It has an additional role in identifying a subgroup of patients, with nonerosive arthritis, Raynaud's phenomenon, and 'machinist's hands'. The most distinctive feature, however, is the high prevalence of ILD in this subgroup. The severity of the lung involvement does not correlate with the titre of anti-Jo-1 antibody.

Several new MSAs have recently been described. For example, anti-KL6 antibody has emerged as a useful marker of activity of ILD. However, many of the autoantibody assays are only available in research laboratories.

**Table 5.13 Syndromes associated with myositis-specific antibodies**

### Anti-Jo-1 (antihistidyl-tRNA synthetase) antibodies

Myositis in younger age group

Often acute onset

Interstitial lung disease (80% if Jo-1)

Nonerosive arthritis

Raynaud's phenomenon

### Anti-signal recognition peptide antibodies

Acute onset of severe myositis, necrotizing disease histologically

*Often autumn onset*

Higher incidence of dysphagia

Lower incidence of interstitial lung disease

Steroid resistance

### Anti-Mi-2 antibodies

Dermatomyositis, with prominent cutaneous involvement

Better treatment outcomes

### Anti-CADM-140 antibodies

Specific for clinically amyopathic dermatomyositis

Acute interstitial lung disease

### Anti-p155/p140 antibodies

Dermatomyositis, especially associated with malignancy

### Myositis-associated autoantibodies

The MAAs are generally seen in overlap syndromes. Anti-PM-Scl is seen in the scleroderma–myositis overlap, which has been termed 'scleromyositis', where the scleroderma has limited cutaneous features, mild myositis, and a good response to treatment. Anti-snRNPs (for example, anti-U1RNP) are associated with overlapping CTD, such as Reynaud's, dactylitis, SLE, and arthritis. These autoantibodies are useful for the diagnosis and classification of IIM. They play a role in predicting the course of disease and response to treatment and are an expanding field of research.

### Electromyography

EMG is an essential component of the diagnostic work-up, as 90% of patients with active myositis have an abnormal EMG (*Table 5.14*). It confirms the disease process to be myopathic, but may also confirm muscle involvement in those who present only with systemic or cutaneous features. If muscle involvement is patchy, testing of multiple sites is required, and may reveal disease limited to the paraspinal muscles. As symmetrical disease is a hallmark of IIM, EMG can also be used to identify a contralateral muscle to biopsy. The normal muscle should be electrically silent at rest, with no action potentials. Certain disease states show spontaneous muscle activity when at rest. Often these potentials have abnormal morphology: of most diagnostic significance is the presence of fibrillation potentials. Damaged myocyte fibres that have lost their innervations produce characteristic positive fibrillation potentials (**5.12**).

Interpretation of EMG is not straightforward. In normal muscle, introduction of the EMG needle may stimulate some brief spontaneous activity. However, pronounced 'insertional activity' is a feature of IIM. Spontaneous myotonic discharges are not specific. Complex repetitive

discharges indicate primary muscle disease and are often associated with chronic disease. Active muscle inflammation of myositis may cause intramuscular neuronal inflammation, and myopathic and neuropathic patterns may be seen on the EMG. In severely atrophied muscle, the only finding may be neuropathic.

### Biopsy

Muscle biopsy is the key investigation to establish the diagnosis of inflammatory myopathy and to exclude other causes of muscle weakness, such as degenerative and neurological disease. Where IBM is identified on electron microscopy, response to treatment can also be predicted. Tissue is required from a site with active inflammation, but if the muscle is extensively damage by disease, necrosis and atrophy of the muscle fibres make interpretation of the biopsy difficult. The biopsy must not be taken from a site recently used for EMG, and it is important to choose an appropriate site for biopsy (*Table 5.15*).

The hallmark histological findings are inflammatory features such as perivascular inflammatory cell infiltrate. Myopathic processes cause rounding of the muscle fibre and variation in fibre size. This is associated with necrosis and evidence of phagocytosis. Neuropathic changes in the

| Table 5.14 Typical EMG features suggestive of inflammatory myositis |
| --- |
| Spontaneous fibrillation potentials |
| Prolonged insertional activity |
| Complex repetitive discharges |
| Resting positive sharp waves |
| Short-duration, low-amplitude, complex, polyphasic potentials during muscle contraction |

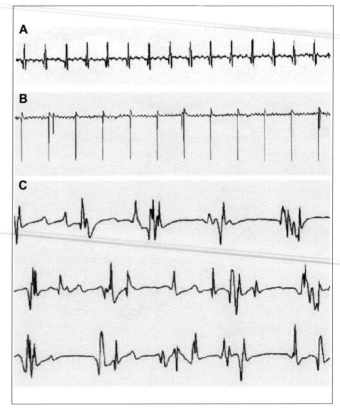

**5.12** Examples of myopathic EMG traces.

**Table 5.15 Choice of biopsy site**

Ideally biopsy proximal muscles – quadriceps and biceps most commonly used

Moderately weak without significant atrophy

Avoid muscles with recent trauma, such as EMG, local anaesthetic and IM injections

Symmetrical disease patterns allow identification of contralateral muscle involvement with EMG/MRI

In patchy disease, MRI is useful in identifying biopsy site

**Table 5.16 Use of different imaging modalities in the assessment of patients with inflammatory myositis**

| Imaging modality | Role |
|---|---|
| Plain film radiology | To demonstrate soft tissue calcification (juvenile dermatomyositis) |
| CT | To differentiate normal from diseased muscle<br>To locate site for muscle biopsy<br>To define muscle bulk |
| Ultrasound | To assess muscle atrophy<br>To provide real time observation of fasciculations |
| MRI | To detect subtle/early changes<br>To locate site for muscle biopsy<br>To provide semiquantitative assessment of disease response to treatment |

muscle tissue (such as angular muscle fibres and distinctive target fibres) are sought to exclude neurological causes for muscle weakness. As well as histological examination, histochemistry, electron microscopy, and enzyme assays are also useful. These tests are important for confirming muscle inflammation, but also for excluding other causes and defining subgroups of disease, such as IBM, which are seen on electron microscopy.

### Imaging

There are numerous imaging modalities for the evaluation of myositis, including plain film radiology, ultrasound, and CT (see *Table 5.16* for comparisons). MRI has emerged as the most useful form of imaging in the assessment of myositis and most often the thighs are studied. Active inflammation is identified by muscle oedema on MRI. In focal disease, there is a role for MRI-guided biopsy to reduce the rates of false-negative results. However, its use may be limited by cost and availability.

## Management of inflammatory myositis

### Induction of remission and maintenance

Corticosteroids are generally accepted as first choice in inflammatory myositis, although evidence from large controlled studies systematically investigating the effect of corticosteroids is lacking. High-dose oral prednisone or intravenous methyl prednisolone pulses followed by lower-dose oral corticosteroids should be administered initially and the corticosteroids tapered according to the effect on CK levels, symptoms and signs such as myalgia and weakness. Prednisone alone may be successful in inducing remission. However, additional immunosuppressive therapy, such as AZA, ciclosporin, MTX, or myco-phenolate mofetil (MMF) may be started in parallel for their steroid-sparing properties and especially in glucocorticoid-resistant disease and those with involvement of heart and lung (*Table 5.17*). There is little evidence from randomized, controlled trials to support this practice but

**Table 5.17 Drugs used in the management of inflammatory myositis (polymyositis)**

| Drug | Main use |
|------|----------|
| Corticosteroids | Induction of remission |
| Azathioprine | Steroid-sparing |
| Ciclosporin | Steroid-sparing |
| Methotrexate | Steroid-sparing |
| Mycophenolate mofetil | Steroid-sparing |
| Cyclophosphamide | Life-threatening disease including cardiac/pulmonary disease |

there have been some reports suggesting benefit as described below.

Cyclophosphamide is used to treat organ- and life-threatening manifestations such as cardiac or pulmonary involvement. Successful treatment with at least six intravenous pulses of cyclophosphamide for ILD in DM/PM with improvement in exercise tolerance, lung function tests, neutrophil reduction in bronchoalveolar lavage fluids, and reduction of HRCT opacities has been reported.

Efficacy of MTX has been demonstrated in retrospective studies, particularly when patients did not respond sufficiently to corticosteroid therapy. No difference was found between MTX and ciclosporin in a small study. A few case reports and case series suggest that ciclosporin is effective in DM- and PM-related ILD. For AZA, a retrospective study showed response rates of 67%, whereas a prospective study could not demonstrate a difference in CK levels of patients treated with corticosteroids and AZA compared to corticosteroids alone after 3 months, but showed a glucocorticoid-sparing effect and reduced disability after 3 years. One study compared the effect of MTX and AZA in patients with incomplete response to corticosteroids and found that MTX may be superior in this setting. Case reports and small case series suggest that MMF may have steroid-sparing effects as well as reducing CK levels and improving muscle strength in inflammatory myositis.

### Biologicals

TNF-antagonists are reported to be effective in a few case reports and case series although there are also reports of unsuccessful administration of the TNF-antagonist etanercept. Rituximab was partially effective in reducing CK and improving muscle strength in two open-label studies with DM patients and a single case report in PM. In summary, the use of biologicals in inflammatory myositis cannot be recommended at present. Biologicals may be taken into consideration in refractory cases but their use needs further evaluation.

## Summary

Inflammatory myositis can be associated with many CTDs. PM and DM are the most common forms of inflammatory myositis. They are characterized by the insidious onset of a symmetrical proximal muscle weakness and systemic features, and well-defined dermatological features define DM. A subgroup of patients have myositis related to an underlying malignancy. Diagnosis requires typical clinical features, high serum levels of muscle enzymes, EMG findings, and histological features of muscle inflammation. Autoantibodies can be used to assist diagnosis, define clinical subgroups, and define prognosis. Corticosteroids are the mainstay of therapy but to prevent long-term side-effects of corticosteroid therapy, additional immuno-suppressants are used for their glucocorticoid-sparing properties. For organ-threatening disease, intravenous cyclophosphamide is the treatment of choice. In less severe cases immunosuppressants such as MTX, ciclosporin, and MMF may be used but none of these therapeutic options are based on randomized controlled studies.

## Further reading

Bohan A, Peter J (1975). Polymyositis and dermatomyositis (first of two parts). *NEJM* **292**:3447.

Dalakas MC, Reinhard H (2003). Polymyositis and dermatomyositis. *Lancet* **362**:971–82.

Targoff IN, Miller FW, Medsger TA Jr, Oddis CV (1997). Classification criteria for the idiopathic inflammatory myopathies. *Curr Opin Rheumatol* **9**:527–35.

Zong M, Lundberg IE (2011). Pathogenesis, classification and treatment of inflammatory myopathies. *Nat Rev Rheumatol* May;7(5):297–306.

# Chapter 6

# Systemic sclerosis

*Philip Clements and Daniel E Furst*

## Definition and pathophysiology

Systemic sclerosis (SSc) usually has, and is defined by, skin involvement but its real impact lies in its major systemic complications. The pathophysiology is thought to be the result of an interplay among three characteristic features: (1) an obliterative vasculopathy that affects many organs; (2) infiltration of collagen (fibrous tissue) into many organs including the skin; and (3) immune activation and inflammation. What the trigger is that initiates the disease is unknown; however, once the disease starts, the manifestations are usually the result of the interplay among the three characteristic features.

## Epidemiology

### Incidence and prevalence

Although the data are surprisingly difficult to obtain, it appears that the incidence of systemic sclerosis in the US is probably between 10 and 20 cases per million population per year. Prevalence is between 140 and 290 cases per million, except in the Choctaw Indians of Oklahoma where it is 3–4 times higher. Internationally a similar incidence and prevalence are found in Australia, but in other populations (such as the UK, Japan, and Iceland), the incidence rate is significantly lower, being between 4 and 6 new cases per million per year, with a prevalence of between 30 and 70 cases per million.

### Effect of ethnicity and gender on the disease

In African-American women the percentage of patients with diffuse disease is approximately 70% compared to 30% with limited disease; this frequency is inverted in most Caucasian populations, being approximately 30%

with diffuse disease and 70% with limited disease. Except in Choctaw Indians (where the prevalence of SCL-70 is 70%) the prevalence of SCL-70 positivity is approximately 10–20% while anti-centromere positivity ranges up to 35%.

In general, the mortality of SSc is significantly higher in men than women and is higher in African-American women than in Caucasian women.

### Environmental risk factors

Occupational exposures to some solvents, notably trichloroethylene, may be associated with a slightly increased probability of developing SSc (odds ratio of about 3) but no clear association has been made with silica dust or other environmental exposures. On the other hand, exposure to unadulterated (rapeseed) cooking oil and to tainted L-tryptophan have been associated with outbreaks of scleroderma-like disease.

### Genetic factors

There are HLA associations with anti-centromere antibodies, anti-SCL-70, anti-U1-RNP, anti-PM-SCL and antifibrillarin RNA polymerases, although these represent a large range of specific HLA associations (e.g. DR B1*01,*04,*08;DGB1*0401,*0501,*0302, etc.). Non-HLA gene associations with tumour growth factor- (TGF-) beta, fibrillin, fibronectin and secreted protein, acidic and rich in cysteine (SPARC) have been found but remain somewhat controversial. Recently, the PTPN22 change has been associated with both susceptibility and protection from SSc, depending upon a specific allele. Relationships with TGF-beta and SPARC genes seem most likely. Overall, these associations often include those involving the extracellular matrix, vascular response, and immunity, although involvement of other pathways is also sometimes found.

Microchimerism is the presence of a small number of cells in an individual that originate from another individual and therefore are genetically distinct from the cells of the host individual. While still somewhat unclear, there appears to be a relationship between microchimerism and SSc, raising the possibility that microchimerism, most likely involving the passage of cells from one or more fetuses into the maternal circulation, may be operative in the pathogenesis of SSc.

## Presentation and assessment of systemic sclerosis

This multisystem disease usually presents with typical skin and vascular manifestations but the prognosis is associated with the amount and severity of internal organ involvement.

### Skin manifestations

Skin involvement gives the disorder its common name, 'scleroderma' or hard skin. Rodnan proposed that the skin involvement has three phases: (1) oedematous, (2) indurative, and (3) atrophic.

The first phase (oedematous) has the clinical appearance of being 'puffy' or swollen (**6.1, 6.2**). Although the phase is called oedematous, there is very little in the way of true 'pitting oedema' as the oedema is interstitial. The second phase (indurative) is the first phase that is truly characteristic of sclerosis of the skin (**6.3, 6.4**). In this phase the skin is often 'hard' to the touch; a biopsy will usually show increased bundles of young collagen infiltrating the dermis and crowding out hair follicles and sweat and oil glands. The observer may not be able to pinch the skin to

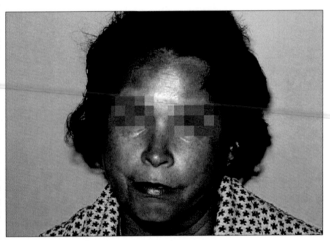

**6.1** Puffy face (oedematous) in SSc.

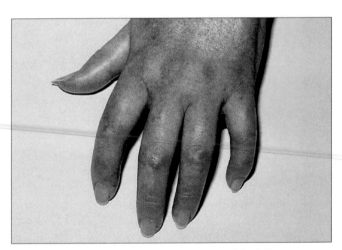

**6.2** Puffy hand and fingers (oedematous) in SSc.

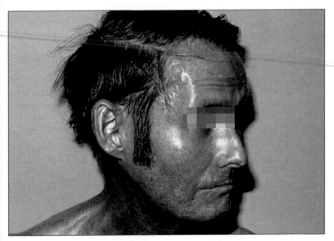

**6.3** Indurated face in SSc.

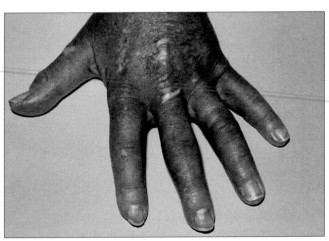

**6.4** Indurated hand in SSc.

make a skin fold. In this phase the skin is said to be 'thick and tight'. The first and second phases may imperceptibly blend together very early in the course of the disease.

The thickening process will plateau. There will then be a phase in which the excess collagen disappears from the dermis (probably the collagen is reabsorbed) and the skin 'thins'. This is the third phase (atrophy) (**6.5, 6.6**). In the atrophic phase the skin may return to its predisease thickness or it may become thinner than normal (the dermis in particular). Often in this phase the thinned skin may stay tethered to the underlying muscle, bone, and subcutaneous tissues, and the clinician may not be able to pinch the skin into a skin fold. In this case, the skin is said to be 'thin and tight'.

### Skin scoring

Although the skin is the largest organ in the body, it is not in a localized area, like the lungs or the heart. Rather it is spread all over the outside of the body. This has made it difficult to assess skin involvement quantitatively. Rodnan pioneered a methodology that sampled multiple areas of skin that are likely to be involved in SSc. The earliest clinical manifestation of skin involvement is usually thickness. Rodnan proposed a method in which the trained observer estimates skin thickness (the method is not meant to measure tethering) on a 0–4 scale by clinical palpation. The present modification assesses thickness on a 0–3 scale in 17 body areas (**6.7**). In Figure **6.8** the examining fingers pinch a normal skin fold on the middle phalanx of the

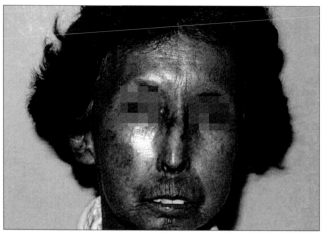

**6.5** Atrophic face in SSc.

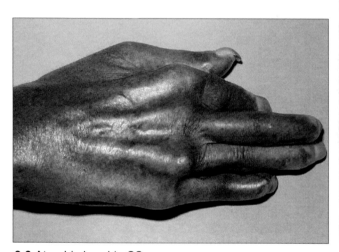

**6.6** Atrophic hand in SSc.

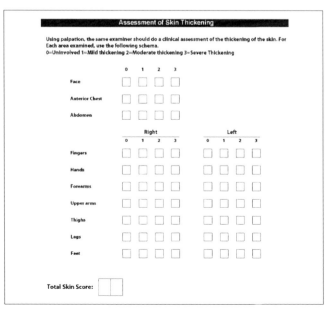

**6.7** Skin score sheet.

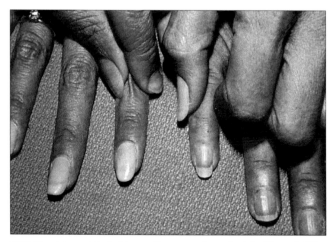

**6.8** Pinching skin folds on fingers of control (left) and SSc (right) patients.

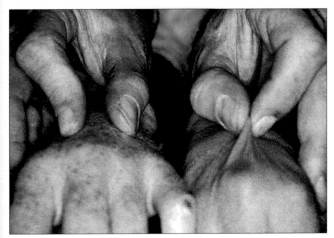

**6.9** Pinching skin folds on hands of SSc (left) and control (right) patients.

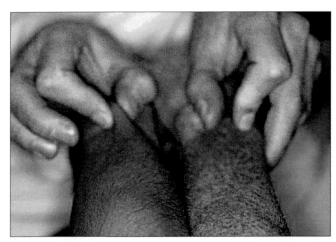

**6.10** Pinching skin folds on forearms of control (left) and SSc (right) patients.

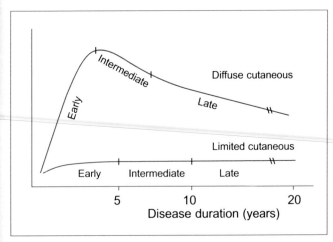

**6.11** Course of skin score over time.

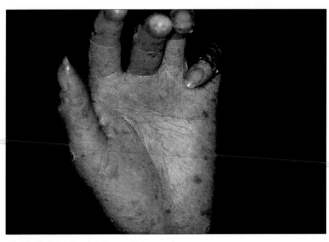

**6.12** Telangiectasias of the palm.

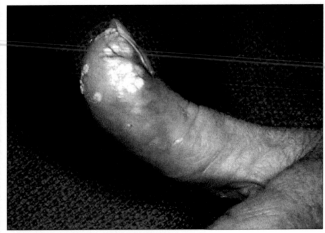

**6.13** Calcinosis of the thumb.

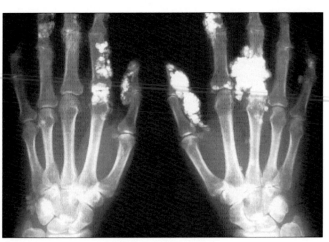

**6.14** Calcinosis on X-ray of the hands.

control finger but they cannot pinch the skin into a fold in the same area of the SSc finger. The examining fingers also assess thickness (not shown). Figures **6.9** and **6.10** also show normal folds in control subjects and the inability to pinch thick sclerodermatous skin into folds in SSc subjects. The assessments of thickness on the 0–3 scale are then recorded on to a skin scoring sheet (**6.7**).

Assessing skin thickness using the modified Rodnan skin score over time is useful in documenting the course of skin involvement over time, in the clinic, and in treatment trials. The extent of skin thickening has led to a division of patients into those who have extensive, widespread, or diffuse skin thickening or involvement (skin thickening proximal, as well as distal, to the elbows and knees, with or without facial involvement) and those who have distal or limited skin involvement (skin thickening distal but not proximal to the elbows and knees, with or without facial involvement). The courses of skin thickness scores for the average patient are shown for limited and for diffuse cutaneous scleroderma (**6.11**). In this diagram the skin score in the limited group remains fairly low and unchanging over many years. In the diffuse group, however, the skin score rapidly increases over the first few years, usually reaching its maximum within 1–3 years of SSc onset, defined as the first sign or symptom typical of SSc other than Raynaud's. The skin score then plateaus for 1–2 years (on average), and then slowly declines as the skin thins, although tethering may remain after thickness subsides. This is the average course; some subjects may have a foreshortened course of thickening/thinning that is months/years shorter than the average while in others the skin may not soften for several years.

### Other skin characteristics

*Telangiectasias* begin to appear within the first several years and by themselves have no prognostic value. They appear as ovals or 'cherry-point' collections of blood vessels primarily on the face, chest, and fingers, although they can also be seen on the torso and on the extremities (**6.5**, **6.12**).

Although *subcutaneous calcinosis* may occur in up to 40% of SSc patients at 10 years, it rarely occurs before the fifth year of SSc. Sometimes the calcinosis is obvious (**6.13**) and at other times it is picked up serendipitously on X-ray (**6.14**). Calcinosis is most commonly seen in the hands, but may also be seen in the subcutaneous tissues of virtually any area of the body (see **6.26**).

*Digital pitting scars* are secondary to ischaemic disease of the fingers. They are permanent 'divots' in the fingertips (**6.15**, **6.16**). They should be distinguished from active digital tip ulcers, some of which heal slowly without leaving a permanent divot while others leave a permanent divot. Digital pitting scars are rarely seen in other disorders.

*Contractures of the joints* probably result from fibrosis of the skin and of the joint capsule, tendon sheaths, and ligaments around the joints. The most common contractures are of the fingers (80–90% of patients with scleroderma); the most severe finger contractures usually occur in the diffuse SSc variant (**6.17**). Contractures of larger joints are more commonly seen in diffuse SSc and can include wrist, elbow, shoulder, hips, knees, and ankles.

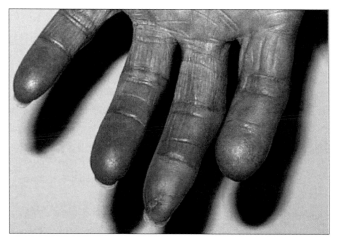

**6.15** Digital pitting scar with Raynaud's phenomenon.

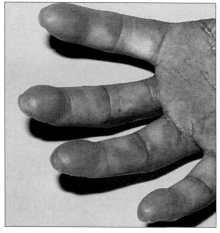

**6.16** Digital pitting ulcers.

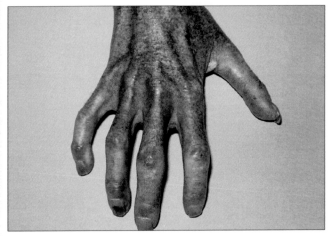

**6.17** Finger contractures in scleroderma.

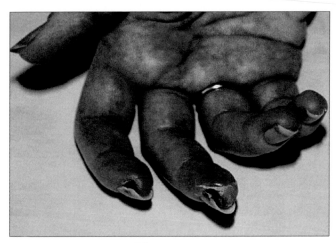

**6.18** Digit tip ulcers in SSc.

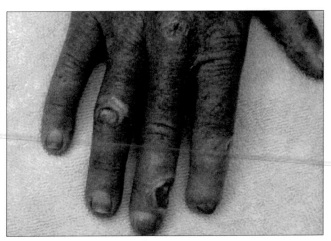

**6.19** Other types of hand and finger ulcers in a patient with absent ulnar artery pulsations.

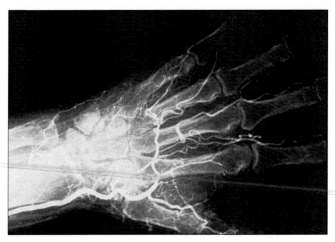

**6.20** Absence of the ulnar artery on angiogram.

### Vascular involvement

*Raynaud's phenomenon* occurs in about 90% of SSc patients (diffuse and limited alike). Raynaud's episodes in SSc often demonstrate only two of the three colour changes that may be seen in Raynaud's in response to cold or emotion: blue/purple and white. The third colour, red, rarely occurs in SSc, as it represents reflex vasodilatation that often is absent in the vessels that are affected by adventitial and intimal thickening in SSc. The tip of the middle finger in Figure **6.15** shows purplish discoloration in addition to the digital pitting scar.

*Ischaemic disease* (cutaneous ulcers, particularly in the fingers) is frequent, particularly in cold climates and cold weather. Ischaemic ulcers of the fingertips are seen (**6.18**), and digital ulcers in other locations can also occur (**6.19**). In some instances these areas of digital necrosis may signal vascular obstruction, particularly of the ulnar artery (**6.20**).

Nailfold capillaroscopy has become a very useful confirmatory test for patients who present an atypical picture of 'scleroderma'. The vascular abnormalities are quite characteristic when present and should be looked for

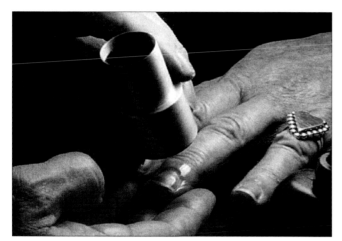

**6.21** Performing 'poor man's' capillaroscopy.

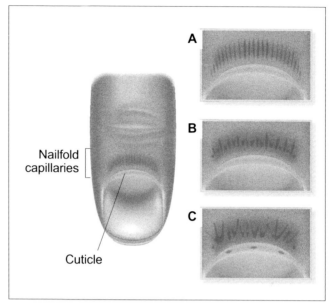

**6.22** Diagram to illustrate nailfold capillary abnormalities seen on capillaroscopy. **A**: Normal nailfold capillaries, like a 'picket-fence'; **B**: mild SSc with abnormally configured and dilated capillaries; **C**: more severe SSc with markedly abnormal configurations and dilatation of capillaries, with 'drop-out' or loss of the number of capillaries and with cuticle haemorrhages ('rust coloured' deposits in the cuticle).

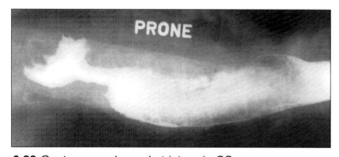

**6.23** Gastro-oesophageal stricture in SSc.

in confusing cases. A simple method uses readily available lubricant jelly to coat the distal finger just proximal to the cuticle. A magnifying lens (an ophthalmoscope can be used but may not provide as clear a view as the use of a 10× microscope eyepiece [**6.21**] or of a Dermatoscope™) can then be used to view the nailfold capillaries ('poor man's' capillaroscopy). A sample of normal capillaries is compared to a sample of typical abnormalities in Figure **6.22**. The most typical SSc abnormalities include capillary drop-out and increased vessel size and architectural distortions of the vessel.

### Gastrointestinal involvement

*Oesophageal involvement* is present in more than 80% of SSc patients. The primary defect is in the vasanervorum of the intestinal smooth muscle. This results in hypomotility and decreased contractility of the enteric smooth muscle with loss of normal peristalsis. This involvement may result in the sensation of dysphagia but also in gastro-oesophageal reflux disease (GERD). Acid reflux may then lead to gastro-oesophageal stricture (**6.23**). With or without stricture, there may be oesophageal dilatation that can be seen in a chest X-ray or computed tomography (CT) scan of the chest.

*Gastric involvement* may lead to gastric atony and retention and to gastroantral vascular ectasia (watermelon stomach) (**6.24**). The *small intestine* also may be involved. Duodenal dilatation is frequent and may be seen on an upper GI barium study (**6.25**). In more serious instances, the bowel may become so hypotonic that intestinal pseudo-obstruction may occur (**6.25**). *Large intestinal involvement* may result in dilated colon, constipation, and intestinal pseudo-obstruction. Rectal hypomotility may result in faecal incontinence and rectal prolapse.

### Lung (interstitial and pulmonary vascular) involvement

*Interstitial lung disease* (ILD) is typified by reduced lung physiology (reduced forced vital capacity [FVC] and total lung capacity) without obstructive characteristics. Although interstitial change can be seen on plain chest X-ray (**6.26**), chest high-resolution computed tomography (HRCT) (**6.27**) is a more sensitive tool for finding interstitial changes (i.e. ground-glass opacification, fibrosis, traction bronchiectasis, and honeycombing) that mark the patient likely to have progressive ILD.

*Pulmonary vascular disease* is typified by a declining diffusing capacity for carbon monoxide ($DL_{CO}$) relative to the FVC, exercise-induced pulmonary hypertension in the face of normal resting pulmonary pressures (on echocardiogram and right heart catheterization), and resting pulmonary arterial hypertension (PAH). In its later stages its effects may been seen on a chest X-ray, showing cardiomegaly with an accentuated pulmonary outflow tract on the left side of the heart shadow and/or an enlarged pulmonary outflow tract on the right side of the heart (**6.28**). The echocardiogram may show an elevated right ventricular systolic pressure (measured from the tricuspid outflow jet) and dilated right ventricular and/or atrial dimensions as the result of chronically elevated right heart pressures (**6.29**). While the echocardiogram is used by many as a screening tool, the echocardiogram frequently cannot produce a measurement of right ventricular systolic pressure (RVSP), or over-reads the RVSP. As a result, a right heart catheterization should be performed to document right-sided pressures.

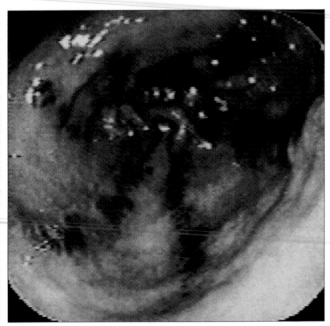

**6.24** 'Watermelon stomach' in SSc.

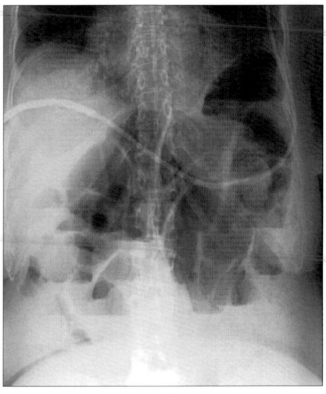

**6.25** Dilated intestine with air-fluid levels.

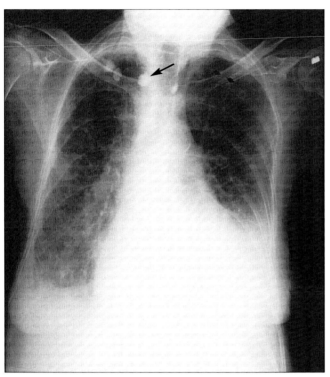

**6.26** ILD seen on chest X-ray. The arrow points to subcutaneous calcinosis.

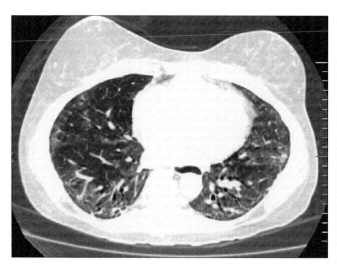

**6.27** ILD by HRCT (ground-glass opacification and fibrosis, most likely from non-specific interstitial pneumonitis [NSIP]).

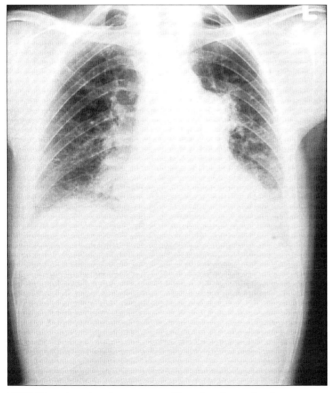

**6.28** Prominent pulmonary outflow tract on chest X-ray in PAH.

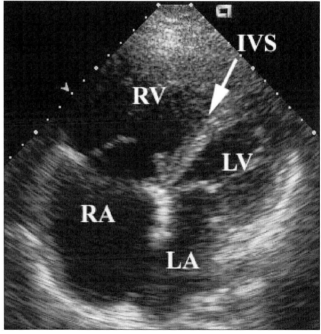

**6.29** Echocardiogram of PAH (dilated right ventricle and atrium and flattening of interventricular septum). IVS, interventricular septum; LA, left atrium; LV, left ventricle; RA, right atrium; RV, right ventricle.

### Renal involvement

The underlying pathology in the kidneys is vascular in nature. Even in the absence of 'renal crisis' (defined as renal failure, usually but not always in the presence of accelerated hypertension), there is a progressive vasculopathy characterized by intimal proliferation that progressively obliterates the vascular lumen. This occurs especially in the arcuate and interlobular arteries in the corticomedullary junction and renal cortex (**6.30**). This is similar to the vasculopathy that is seen throughout the body (i.e. digital arteries and pulmonary arterioles for example). This leads to a general reduction in renal blood flow and a gradually progressive but mild loss of glomerular function over time.

Renal crisis, on the other hand, is a process that suddenly involves the afferent arteriole with thrombotic microangiopathy and fibrinoid necrosis and ischaemia of the juxtaglomerular apparatus and the glomerulus itself (**6.30**). The release of renin leads to activation of angiotensin II, and that results in the features recognized as renal crisis. Untreated this will lead to cortical necrosis and death of the glomerulus, permanent renal failure, and death of the patient (80+% mortality within 1 year of onset of renal crisis). Management with angiotensin-converting enzyme inhibitors (ACEIs) usually dramatically alters the outcome in a positive way.

### Cardiac involvement

Cardiac involvement may affect the pericardium, the myocardium, and the conduction system.

*Pericardial involvement* is most often manifested with moderate or large effusion (**6.31** shows an enlarged heart shadow). This can be confirmed with an echocardiogram or chest CT, which can help distinguish effusion from dilatation of the ventricles. The HRCT of the chest in Figure **6.32** shows a large collection of pericardial fluid anterior and lateral to the heart. Myocardial involvement may also manifest as an enlarged heart shadow (**6.33**). In this case the echocardiogram may show reduced ventricular systolic performance (reduced ejection fraction).

*Conduction system abnormalities and arrhythmias* are very frequent when routinely screened for. Clinically significant arrhythmias are less frequent and are usually supraventricular in origin. Some patients do have ventricular arrhythmias (bursts of ventricular tachycardia are shown in **6.34**) and some may develop heart block. Figure **6.33** shows the chest X-ray of a patient with an enlarged heart shadow from low output ventricular function and a pacemaker that was installed to control her SSc-induced heart block.

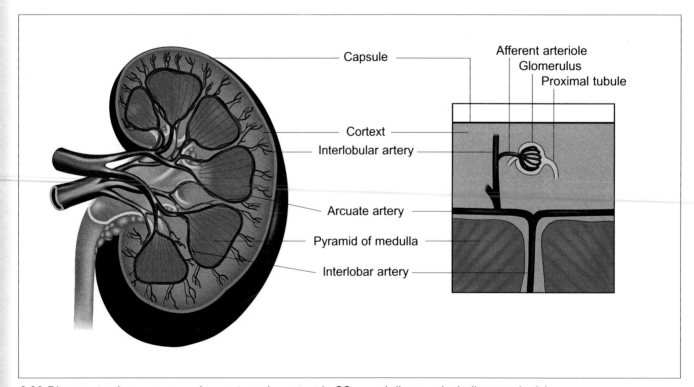

**6.30** Diagram to show renovascular anatomy important in SSc renal disease, including renal crisis.

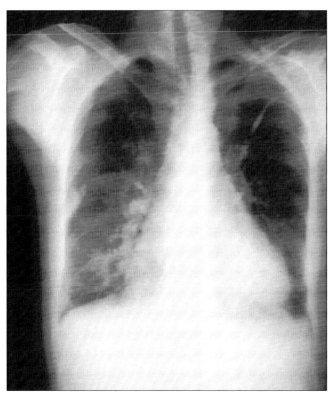

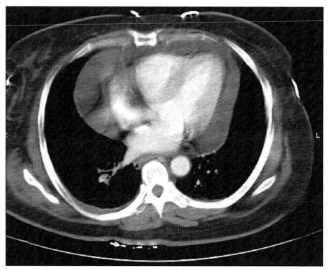

**6.32** Large anterior pericardial effusion on chest HRCT (grey area anterior and lateral to heart shadow).

**6.31** Pericardial effusion on chest X-ray.

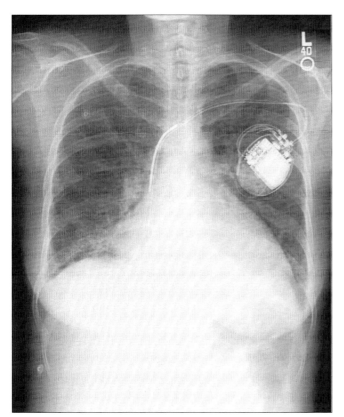

**6.33** Low cardiac output secondary cardiomyopathy and implanted pacemaker to control SSc-induced heart block.

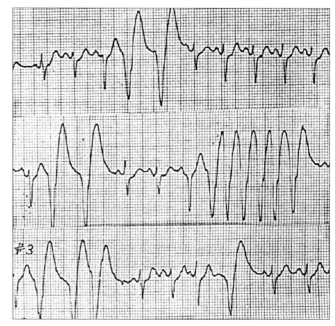

**6.34** Bursts of ventricular tachycardia on ECG.

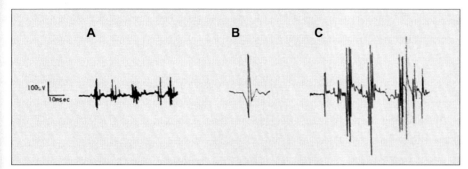

**6.35** EMG action potentials for (**A**) polymyositis, (**B**) healthy control, and (**C**) myopathy.

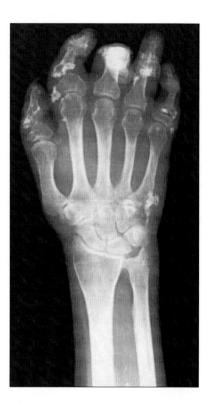

**6.36** X-ray showing joint space loss in the wrist and second metacarpophalangeal joint, digit tuft and phalangeal resorption, subcutaneous calcinosis, and loss of the normal soft tissue convexity on the ulnar side of the hand.

## Musculoskeletal involvement

*Muscle involvement* most typically results from a noninflammatory myopathy that does not require steroids or immunosuppressives; less frequently muscle weakness results from an inflammatory myositis that does require steroids and/or immunsuppressives (~5%). Exceptionally high serum creatine phosphokinase levels (≥10 times the upper limit of normal [ULN]), electromyographic (EMG) abnormalities (low amplitude, polyphasic motor unit potentials, coupled with signs of denervation) and muscle biopsy (showing inflammatory infiltrates, muscle necrosis, and regeneration) most clearly substantiate the presence of true inflammatory myositis (**6.35**). In Figure **6.35**, EMG myopotentials that suggest noninflammatory myopathy (polyphasic motor unit potentials without denervation and often of normal amplitude) and inflammatory myositis are compared to those seen in a patient with normal muscle unit action potentials.

*Skeletal involvement* may manifest as tender (and sometimes swollen) joints, tendonitis (with or without friction rubs), and bursitis. The most classic findings on hand X-ray are subcutaneous calcinosis (**6.14, 6.36**), loss of the normal concave appearance of the soft tissues on the ulnar side of the hand (**6.14, 6.20, 6.36**) and digit tuft resorption (**6.36**). In some instances there may also be joint space narrowing, marginal erosions, and other evidence of true inflammatory joint disease (**6.36**), which may be suggestive of, but not typical of, rheumatoid arthritis.

## Management of systemic sclerosis

Even though several hypotheses have been proposed to explain the causation of SSc, none of these hypotheses has led to a cure, nor for that matter have they produced a treatment that modifies the ultimate course of SSc (with one or two exceptions). Thus there are no cures that will be discussed, nor will there be a discussion of treatments which modify the disease (with the exception of ACEIs in the management of renal crisis). Since the treatments that are available are largely organ specific in nature, our discussion will be directed at the treatment of organ-based involvements.

### Treatment of cutaneous manifestations

The extent and degree of skin thickening often determines the need, or not, for treatment of skin thickening. Those with diffuse skin involvement and high skin scores (especially skin scores >20 out of a maximum of 51) are the patients most likely to become disabled, to lose motion of small and large joints from contractures, to develop cardiac and heart involvement, to complain of polyarthritic joint pain, and to die prematurely. Thus multiple studies have been undertaken in patients with high skin scores to find a treatment that can improve their lot.

To date only two treatments have been shown in randomized controlled trials (RCTs) to be effective in decreasing skin thickening and improving global assessment by patient and/or physician: methotrexate (MTX) and cyclophosphamide (CYC). In early diffuse patients with high skin scores, oral MTX can be administered weekly, beginning with doses of 15 mg weekly (supplemented with folic acid 1 mg daily), titrated upward to 25 mg weekly over several months. A significant response should not be expected until 6–9 months of MTX, and MTX should be continued for at least 1 year. In patients who have attained skin scores of ≥25–30 in the first 12–18 months, and/or have continued to progress in spite of 3–6 months of MTX, CYC may be administered. Although CYC can be given orally (at a dose of approximately 2 mg/kg/day), CYC by the intravenous route may be preferable. IV CYC can be administered in doses of 500–750 mg/m$^2$ monthly for 6–12 months. Although no RCT has looked at what to do following CYC therapy, additional immunosuppressive therapy (MTX or mycophenolate mofetil [MMF]) is probably warranted and may be continued for months to years (i.e. until the skin score drops to a low level or to a level that the patient considers acceptable and/or stable).

### Management of vascular features

Mild but tolerable Raynaud's may require nothing more than keeping warm. Patients who experience very symptomatic Raynaud's or who have developed cutaneous ulcers or necrotic digits may benefit from several types of vasodilators (given individually or together): calcium-channel blockers (CCBs) of the dihydropyridine class (i.e. nifedipine, amlodipine, isradapine, felodipine); topical nitroglycerin (NTG); phosphodiesterase-5 inhibitors (PDE-5 inhibitors: sildenafil, tildenafil); parenteral prostacyclin infusions (epoprostenol, treprostinil, or iloprost); and endothelin receptor antagonists (ERA: bosentan). Symptomatic Raynaud's (particularly with ulcerations or necrosis) may require a CCB, such as nifedipine XL 30–120 mg daily as the first choice. If there is an inadequate response or adverse event with nifedipine, switching to another medication in the dihydropyridine class is reasonable. Sildenafil 20–50 mg tid or tildenafil 10 mg qd may also be beneficial. Topical NTG ointment 2% may be applied circumferentially around the proximal 2/3 of a critically ischaemic fingertip 3–4 times a day for at least 20–30 minutes. Topical NTG ointment and PDE-5 inhibitors (sildenafil, tildenafil) have a significant adverse interaction and should not be used together. Critically ischaemic digits may require IV or subcutaneous prostacyclin (epoprostenol or treprostinil, which are approved for treating PAH) on a 24 hours/7 days a week basis (dosed up to tolerance) for several weeks to months to

control. Patients who have a history of recurrent multiple digit ulcers may benefit from the use of an ERA such as bosentan 125 mg bid, which appears to prevent new ulcers, although it has no benefit for healing ulcers already present or for ameliorating the symptoms of Raynaud's (i.e. numbness, pain, tingling).

### Treatment of gastrointestinal complications

Although oesophageal hypomotility with its attendant reflux and dysphagia is the most frequent evidence of GI involvement, the entire GI tract may become involved. The initial lesion in GI tract involvement is hypomotility associated with weak and atrophic smooth muscles in the GI tract, which then leads to a variety of interconnected GI symptoms. Initial treatment of reflux is usually with proton-pump inhibitors (PPI) at least once if not twice a day. They may be supplemented with metoclopramide or erythromycin, which stimulate GI motility in the stomach, and which can reduce symptoms of reflux and postprandial bloating. Resistant delay in gastric emptying has been treated experimentally with gastric pacing, with some apparent success. Persistent vomiting and/or postprandial bloating are often related to gastro-oesophageal stricture, gastric retention, or small-bowel hypomotility with varying degrees of intestinal pseudo-obstruction. Oesophago-gastroduodenostomy (EGD) may be warranted for sorting out these complaints. Dilatation of the gastro-oesophageal junction may be helpful for strictures. Small intestinal bacterial overgrowth (SIBO) may lead to postprandial bloating and/or frequent stools or diarrhoea. If SIBO is suspected, a hydrogen-breath test using oral lactulose (or equivalent) may corroborate the diagnosis of SIBO. Alternatively sequential rotation of 10–14 day courses of broad-spectrum antibiotics (i.e. ciprofloxacin, rifaximin, metronidazole, doxycycline, amoxicillin) may be tried empirically, as may intermittent therapy. If diarrhoea and/or bloating improve, the diagnosis is likely. Several different antibiotics should be tried in succession to find ones that can be continued in rotation for managing SIBO. Constipation may be treated with polyethylene glycol 3350 (Miralax™).

### Management of interstitial lung disease

Before making the diagnosis of SSc-ILD, a HRCT of the chest should confirm that the patient has fibrotic changes, with or without ground-glass opacities. If HRCT changes (particularly fibrotic change) are present, the FVC has fallen below 75% predicted, the patient has had SSc for less than 4–6 years, and the patient reports dyspnoea on exertion (e.g. climbing stairs), CYC may be appropriate, as it is the only treatment that has been shown in two RCTs to slow fibrosis and preserve FVC. CYC can be given in the same dosage regimens as noted above. Once CYC is completed, the patient should continue on oral azathioprine or MMF for several years.

### Management of pulmonary vascular disease

ILD and pulmonary vascular disease (PVD) frequently coexist and therefore the cause of dyspnoea may be difficult to determine. Several cardiac/pulmonary vascular causes of dyspnoea should be investigated: restrictive pulmonary disease, PAH, left ventricular diastolic dysfunction, left ventricular systolic heart failure, pulmonary venous occlusive disease, and pulmonary emboli, for example. The echocardiogram may be a useful screening device but the gold standard for evaluating this difficult situation and for sorting out which cause(s) are resulting in dyspnoea is right heart catheterization. PAH (in isolation or with ILD) is now treatable, with six medications approved by the Food and Drug Administration for PAH in the US: epoprostenol, treprostinil, sildenafil, inhaled iloprost, bosentan, and ambrisentan. Before starting such PAH medication it is imperative that the patient undergoes right heart catheterization to confirm the diagnosis and to exclude all the other possible cardiac, pulmonary, and pulmonary–vascular causes of dyspnoea.

### Management of renal involvement

The prime cause of chronic renal insufficiency is chronically reduced renal perfusion. However, the primary manifestation that requires treatment (and then emergently) is scleroderma renal crisis (SRC): acute, oliguric renal failure, usually associated with accelerated hypertension. Untreated this complication leads to death within 1 year in over 80% of patients. Treatment with ACEIs results in >70% survival at 1 year, and if the patient lives 1 year they are likely to live 5 or more years. Angiotensin-receptor blockers (ARBs) can be added to ACEIs, but ACEIs should be the drugs used first in the management of SRC. Control of blood pressure is the first priority: serum creatinine may continue to rise for several weeks, but then frequently begins to decline. Although some patients progress to dialysis, it is reassuring that >50% of the patients who begin dialysis will be able to come off dialysis within 18 months and will never require dialysis again. ACEIs and/or ARBs should be continued for life regardless of whether the patient is on dialysis or not. Since there is evidence that prednisone in doses of >7.5–15 mg daily or equivalent may be associated with precipitation of SRC (particularly in patients with diffuse scleroderma), caution should be used in using corticosteroids in patients with early diffuse SSc.

### Management of cardiac involvement

Large pericardial effusions are usually harbingers of renal crisis and of themselves do not usually cause tamponade or need primary treatment. Rarely tamponade can occur and may require aspiration and/or a pericardial window. Occasionally pericarditis is inflammatory and steroids or nonsteroidal anti-inflammatory drugs will be required. Cardiac failure should be treated in a conventional manner using diuretics, ACEIs, and digoxin. Arrhythmias should be treated in standard fashion. Persistent symptomatic arrhythmias can be treated medically with anti-arrhythmic drugs and/or ablation if appropriate. Heart block may require an implanted pacemaker.

### Treatment of musculoskeletal features
#### Myositis

True inflammatory myositis requires steroids and immuno-suppressives, as might be used in persons with idiopathic myositis. Noninflammatory myopathy is usually mild but in some cases may lead to significant muscle weakness. There is no specific therapy that can or should be directed at this noninflammatory myopathy. Active muscle strengthening exercises should be encouraged (with physical therapy and/or at home) with either type of muscle involvement.

#### Musculoskeletal pain

Musculoskeletal pain is very common. It can present as a true arthritis, but more commonly presents as a mix of arthritis, tendonitis, bursitis, nonspecific muscle and soft tissue pain, and in 10–15% as fibromyaglia. Low-dose prednisone (≤7.5 mg/day) is often employed for these painful musculoskeletal problems and, if effective, may be continued at low-dose for pain control, keeping in mind the previous caution regarding the use of corticosteroids in patients with diffuse SSc. A few patients with inflammatory polyarthritis may benefit from MTX and/or leflunomide therapy.

# Further reading

Au K, Khanna D, Clements PJ, *et al.* (2009). Current concepts in disease-modifying therapy for systemic sclerosis-associated interstitial lung disease: lessons from clinical trials. *Curr Rheumatol Rep* **11**(2):111–19.

Charles C, Clements P, Furst DE (2006). Systemic sclerosis: hypothesis-driven treatment strategies. *Lancet* **367**(9523):1683–91.

Clements PJ, Roth MD, Elashoff R, *et al.* (2007). Scleroderma lung study (SLS): differences in the presentation and course of patients with limited versus diffuse systemic sclerosis. *Ann Rheum Dis* **66**(12):1641–7.

Herrick A (2008). Diagnosis and management of scleroderma peripheral vascular disease. *Rheum Dis Clin North Am* **34**(1):89–114.

Herrick AL (2008). Systemic sclerosis: an update for clinicians. *Br J Hosp Med (Lond)* **69**(8):464–70.

Kowal-Bielecka O, Landewe R, Avouac J, *et al.* (2009). EULAR recommendations for the treatment of systemic sclerosis: a report from the EULAR Scleroderma Trials and Research group (EUSTAR). *Ann Rheum Dis* **68**(5):620–8.

Lin AT, Clements PJ, Furst DE (2003). Update on disease-modifying antirheumatic drugs in the treatment of systemic sclerosis. *Rheum Dis Clin North Am* **29**(2):409–26.

Medsger TA, Jr (2003). Natural history of systemic sclerosis and the assessment of disease activity, severity, functional status, and psychologic well-being. *Rheum Dis Clin North Am* **29**(2):255–73.

Steen VD (2003). Scleroderma renal crisis. *Rheum Dis Clin North Am* **29**(2):315–33.

Steen VD (2008). The many faces of scleroderma. *Rheum Dis Clin North Am* **34**(1):1–15.

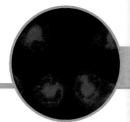
# Chapter 7

# The primary systemic vasculitides

*Wolfgang L Gross and Frank Moosig*

## Definition and classification

In principle vasculitis is either a primary condition or a sequela of another underlying disease. The primary systemic vasculitides (PSV) represent a group of heterogeneous diseases that involve inflammation of blood vessel walls. They are of multifactorial aetiology and their causation remains poorly understood but includes drugs, environmental factors, infections, gender, and other genetic predisposing factors. PSV comprise a broad group of conditions affecting large, medium, or small vessels (*Table 7.1*, *7.1*). Classifications are mostly based on the vessel size.

Definitions for the individual vasculitic syndromes were derived at the Chapel Hill Consensus Conference (CHCC). They provided nomenclature to be used rather than diagnostic or classification criteria and included microscopic polyangiitis (MPA) in contrast to the American College of Rheumatology (ACR) criteria that do not consider MPA or the presence of anti-neutrophil cytoplasmic antibodies (ANCAs).

## Epidemiology of primary systemic vasculitides

### Incidence rates of PSV

Several reports have been published suggesting that the systemic vasculitides have become more common. These studies may reflect increased awareness of these conditions and the more frequent ANCA testing in recent years.

### Table 7.1 Classification of the main disease entities by vessel size and immune phenomena

| Vessel predominantly affected | Vasculitis |
| --- | --- |
| Large arteries | Giant cell arteritis, Takayasu's arteritis |
| Medium arteries | Classical PAN, Kawasaki's disease |
| Small vessels | *Wegener's granulomatosis, Churg–Strauss syndrome, microscopic polyangiitis |
| | **Henoch–Schönlein purpura, cutaneous leukocytoclastic angiitis, cryoglobulinaemia |

*Strongly associated with PR3- or MPO-ANCA in blood; usually no immune complex deposits are seen by immunohistochemistry, therefore termed 'pauci-immune vasculitides'

**Associated with immune complex deposits *in situ*, therefore termed 'immune complex vasculitides'

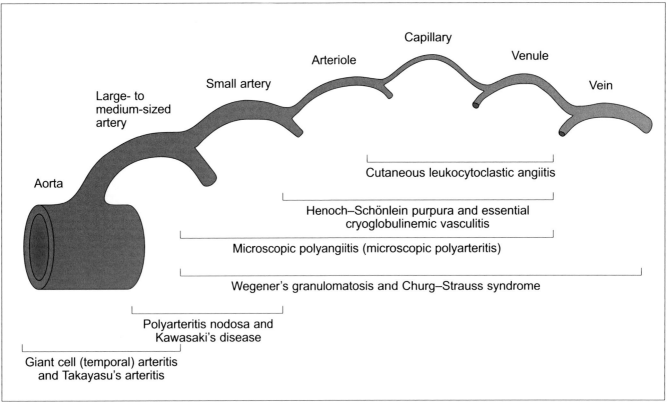

**7.1** Predominant range of vasculitic involvement in PSV. Note that even in the so-called small-vessel vasculitides, medium sized to large arteries might be affected.

However, two large population-based studies in Northern Germany and the UK (Norwich) show stable incidence rates over more than 5 years with only minor fluctuations for all PSV and the individual diseases. *Table 7.2* and Figure **7.2** present data from the largest population-based study, with annual incidence rates for all PSV between 38 and 54/million per year (**7.3**). The incidence rate in Norwich is lower at 19.6/million, though giant cell arteritis (GCA) was not included. Most analyses assessing the epidemiology are derived from Northern Europe, the USA, and Japan. Data from India, Africa, Asia, and South America are not available. Seasonal variations in the onset have been assessed for ANCA-associated vasculitides (AAV) and GCA with no consistent results.

*Giant cell arteritis*
GCA represents the most frequent vasculitis, with incidence rates varying between 15 and 35/100,000 inhabitants in Scandinavia and Olmsted County, USA, in prospective studies of a population aged 50 years and older.

Figures from Germany are lower, with incidence rates of between 3 and 5/100,000 inhabitants. Data from a Japanese study reported incidence rates of about 1.47/100,000. The incidence rates for GCA increase with older age, and women are affected about twice as often as men. The apparent increase in the incidence rates may be related to the population structures.

*Takayasu's arteritis*
Takayasu's arteritis (TA) is rare, with an annual incidence of 1–3/million. TA has been described world-wide and affects women younger than 40 years in most cases.

*Polyarteritis nodosa*
According to the applied criteria incidence rates of polyarteritis nodosa (PAN) vary between 0.4 and 2.0/million in Germany, Spain, and Sweden and 16.0/million in Kuwait (CHCC) and 6–9/million in Norway, Olmsted County, USA, Lithuania, and Norwich, UK (ACR criteria).

**Table 7.2 Incidence rates in a stable and representative population in Northern Germany (2.83 million inhabitants, Schleswig-Holstein) 1998–2006**

| | 1998 | 1999 | 2000 | 2001 | 2002 | 2003 | 2004 | 2005 | 2006 |
|---|---|---|---|---|---|---|---|---|---|
| All PSV | 54 (39;68) | 48 (34;61) | 45 (34;61) | 40 (31;50) | 42 (31;52) | 39 (19; 58) | 38 (25;51) | 38 (25;51) | 54 (39;68) |
| GCA | 17 (8;24) | 9 (3;15) | 9 (3;15) | 10 (4;16) | 13 (6;20) | 13 (6; 20) | 11 (5;18) | 14.2 (7;21) | 17 (8;24) |
| ≥50 yrs | 46 (33;59) | 25 (14;36) | 31 (18;44) | 27 (16;38) | 37 (23;50) | 36 (16;56) | 29 (17;41) | 38 (25;41) | 43 (31;55) |
| ANCA-associated PSV | 11 (5;18) | 9.5 (4;16) | 12 (5;19) | 12 (5;19) | 16 (8;24) | 10 (4;16) | 13.5 (7;20) | 12 (5;19) | 12 (5;19) |
| WG | 8(2;14) | 6 (1;11) | 8 (2;13) | 9 (3;15) | 12 (5;19) | 8 (4;11) | 9 (3;15) | 9 (3;15) | 9 (3;15) |
| MPA | 3 (0;6) | 2.5 (0;6) | 3 (0;6) | 2 (0;4) | 3 (0;6) | 2 (0;4) | 3 (0;6) | 1 (0;3) | 3 (0;6) |
| CSS | 0 | 1 (0;3) | 1.5 (0;3) | 1 (0;3) | 2 (0;4) | 1 (0;3) | 2 (0;4) | 1 (0;3) | 1 (0;3) |
| PAN | 1 (0;3) | 2 (0;4) | 1 (0;2) | 0.4 (0;2) | 0.4 (0;2) | 1 (0;3) | 1.4 (0;2) | 0.4 (0;2) | 1.1 (0;2) |
| HSP | 7 (2;12) | 10 (4;16) | 6 (3;9) | 7 (4;11) | 3 (0;6) | 1 (0;3) | 3 (0;6) | 5 (2;8) | 3.2 (1;6) |
| CLA | 9 (3;15) | 8 (2;14) | 9 (3;15) | 6 (3;9) | 4 (1;7) | 8 (2;14) | 2 (0,4) | 2 (0 ;4) | 9 (3;15) |
| TA | 1 (0;3) | 1 (0;3) | 0.5 (0;2) | 0.4 (0;2) | 0.4 (0;2) | 1 (0;3) | 0.4 (0;2) | 0 | 0.4 (0;2) |
| KD | 0 | 1 (0;3) | 1 (0;2) | 1 (0;3) | 0 | 1 (0;3) | 0 | 1 (0;3) | 1.1 (0;2) |
| UV | 9 (3;15) | 8 (2;14) | 6 (3;9) | 3 (0;6) | 5 (2;8) | 5 (2;8) | 7 (2;12) | 5 (2;8) | 10 (4;16) |

GCA: Giant cell arteritis; WG: Wegener's granulomatosis; MPA: microscopic polyangiitis; CSS: Churg–Strauss syndrome; PAN: polyarteritis nodosa; HSP: Henoch–Schönlein purpura; CLA: cutanous (isolated) leukocytoclastic angiitis; TA: Takayasu's arteritis; KD: Kawasaki's disease; UV: unclassified vasculitis

All new cases per year and per 1 million inhabitants (95% confidence interval)

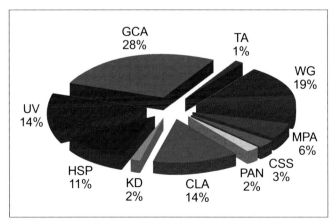

**7.2** Average distribution in Schleswig-Holstein (Germany) between 1998 and 2006. AAV (WG, CSS, MPA) and GCA present with similar incidence rates.

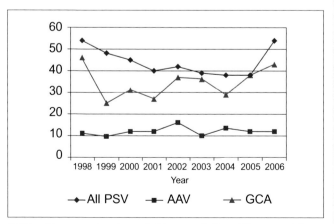

**7.3** Incidence rates in a stable population (Germany) for all PSV, AAV, and GCA 1998–2006.

### ANCA-associated vasculitides

Wegener's granulomatosis (WG) is the most frequent AAV, with an annual incidence of 1–12/million in Europe and the US (Olmsted County, US). Prevalence rates range from 24/million (France) to 131/million (New Zealand). Figures from Germany and Norwich, UK, are similar, with 42/million and 63/million, respectively. The incidence of MPA is less frequent, with figures of between 1/million and 8/million in Europe, 14.8/million in Japan, and 24/million in Kuwait. Incidence rates of Churg–Strauss syndrome (CSS) have been evaluated in Germany, UK, Spain, Olmsted County, USA, and Vilnius, Lithuania, with similar results of 1–4 new cases/year/million and 1–4/million.

### Kawasaki's disease

Kawasaki's disease (KD) presents as mucocutaneous lymph node syndrome complicated by coronariitis in young children between 6 months and 5 years. Annual incidence rates vary geographically with low rates (0–17/100,000 in Europe, the USA, and Australia) and high rates in Japan, China, Hawaii, and West Indies (25–108/100,000).

### Henoch–Schönlein purpura

Henoch–Schönlein purpura (HSP) presents more frequently in patients younger than 17 years (10–20/100,000 in the UK, Spain, Taiwan, and Czech Republic) and with 3–14 cases/million/year in the adult population (Germany, UK, Lithuania, Spain).

### Prevalence of PSV

The prevalence of PSV has been investigated in two areas in Northern and Southern Germany and has shown higher rates in urban populations in both areas, with 220/million in Freiburg and 290/million in Lübeck compared to 171/million and 146/million in the rural areas (Reinhold-Keller *et al.*, 2000) (*Table 7.3*).

## Clinical manifestations and diagnosis of the systemic vasculitides

In this section the PSV will be discussed individually and then the secondary vasculitides will be reviewed more briefly. As described above, the PSV usually are categorized according to the size of the affected vessels. The ACR and the CHCC provided criteria for the classification or definition of these conditions and associated immune phenomena-like autoantibodies (*Table 7.4*).

**Table 7.3 Prevalence rates for GCA, WG, MPA, CSS, and PAN/million inhabitants**

| Vasculitis | Northern Germany 1994 | | Southern Germany 1994 | | France 2000 | Sweden/Lund 2003 (point prevalence) |
|---|---|---|---|---|---|---|
| Population | Urban | Rural | Urban | Rural | Urban | Urban/rural |
| | 217,133 | 232,365 | 198,496 | 227,985 | 1,093,515 | 287,479 |
| GCA | 138 | 39 | 121 | 70 | n.a. | n.a. |
| WG | 55 | 60 | 50 | 35 | 23.7 | 160 |
| MPA | 18 | 0 | 0 0 | | 25.1 | 94 |
| CSS | 14 | 0 | 5 0 | | 10.7 | 14 |
| PAN | 5 | 13 | 5 0 | | 30.7 | 31 |

GCA: Giant cell arteritis; WG: Wegener's granulomatosis; MPA: microscopic polyangiitis; CSS: Churg–Strauss syndrome; PAN: polyarteritis nodosa

**Table 7.4 Names and definitions of vasculitides according to ACR classification criteria and the 1992 CHCC**

## ACR CLASSIFICATION CRITERIA (1)
### Large vessels

*Giant cell arteritis*
1. Development of symptoms or findings beginning at age 50 or older
2. New-onset or new type of localized pain in the head
3. Temporal artery tenderness to palpation or decreased pulsation, unrelated to arteriosclerosis of cervical arteries
4. Erythrocyte sedimentation rate ≥50 mm/hour by the Westergren method
5. Biopsy specimen with artery showing vasculitis characterized by a predominance of mononuclear cell infiltration or granulomatous inflammation, usually with multinucleated giant cells

For purpose of classification, a patient shall be said to have giant cell arteritis if at least three of these five criteria are present

*Takayasu's arteritis*
1. Development of symptoms or findings related to Takayasu's arteritis at age <40 years
2. Development and worsening of fatigue and discomfort in muscles of one or more extremity while in use, especially the upper extremities
3. Decreased pulsation of one or both brachial arteries
4. Difference of >10 mmHg in systolic blood pressure between arms
5. Bruit audible on auscultation over one or both subclavian arteries or abdominal aorta
6. Arteriographic narrowing or occlusion of the entire aorta, its primary branches, or arteries in the proximal upper or lower extremities, not due to arteriosclerosis, fibromuscular dysplasia, or similar causes; changes usually focal or segmental

For classification purpose, a patient shall be said to have Takayasu's arteritis if at least three of these six criteria are present

### Medium vessels

*Polyarteritis nodosa*
1. Loss of 4 kg or more of body weight since illness began, not due to dieting or other factors
2. Mottled reticular pattern over the skin or portions of the extremities or torso
3. Pain and tenderness of the testicles, not due to infection, trauma, or other causes
4. Diffuse myalgias (excluding shoulder and hip girdle) or weakness of muscles or tenderness of leg muscles

## CHCC (2)
### Large vessels

*Giant cell arteritis*
Granulomatous arteritis of the aorta and its major branches, with a predilection for the extracranial branches of the carotid artery. Often involves the temporal artery. Usually occurs in patients older than 50 and often is associated with polymyalgia rheumatica

*Takayasu's arteritis*
Granulomatous inflammation of the aorta and its major branches. Usually occurs in patients younger than 50

### Medium vessels

*Polyarteritis nodosa*
Necrotizing inflammation of medium-sized or small arteries without glomerulonephritis or vasculitis of arterioles, capillaries, or venules

*Continued overleaf*

**Table 7.4** *Continued*

| ACR CLASSIFICATION CRITERIA (1) | CHCC (2) |
|---|---|
| **Medium vessels** | **Medium vessels** |

*Polyarteritis nodosa (continued)*

5. Development of mononeuropathy, multiple mononeuropathy, or polyneuropathy
6. Development of hypertension with diastolic blood pressure higher than 90 mmHg
7. Elevation of BUN >40 mg/dl or creatinine >1.5 mg/dl, not due to dehydration or obstruction
8 Presence of hepatitis B surface antigen or antibody in serum
9. Arteriogram showing aneurysms or occlusions of the visceral arteries,not due to arteriosclerosis, fibromuscular dysplasia, or other noninflammatory causes
10. Histological changes showing the presence of granulocytes or granulocytes and mononuclear leukocytes in the artery wall

For classification purpose, a patient shall be said to have polyarteritis nodosa if at least three of these 10 criteria are present

*Kawasaki's disease*
No definition given by the ACR

*Kawasaki's disease*
Arteritis involving large, medium-sized, and small arteries, and associated with mucocutaneous lymph node syndrome. Coronary arteries are often involved. Aorta and veins may be involved. Usually occurs in children

**Small vessels**

**Small vessels**

*Wegener's granulomatosis*
1. Development of painful or painless oral ulcers or purulent or bloody nasal discharge
2. Chest radiograph showing the presence of nodules, fixed infiltrates or cavities
3. Microhaematuria (>5 red blood cells per high power field) or red cell casts in urine sediment
4. Histological changes showing granulomatous inflammation within the wall of an artery or in the perivascular or extravascular area (artery or arteriole)

For purposes of classification a patient shall be said to have Wegener's granulomatosis if at least two of these four criteria are present

*Wegener's granulomatosis*
Granulomatous inflammation involving the respiratory tract, and necrotizing vasculitis affecting small to medium-sized vessels (e.g. capillaries, venules, arterioles, and arteries). Necrotizing glomerulonephritis is common

*Churg–Strauss syndrome*
1. Asthma: History of wheezing or diffuse high-pitched rales on expiration
2. Eosinophilia: >10% on white blood cell differential count

*Churg–Strauss syndrome*
Eosinophil-rich and granulomatous inflammation involving the respiratory tract, and necrotizing vasculitis affecting

*(Continued)*

**Table 7.4 Continued**

| ACR CLASSIFICATION CRITERIA (1) | CHCC (2) |
|---|---|
| **Small vessels** | **Small vessels** |

*Churg–Strauss syndrome (continued)*

3. History of allergy: History of seasonal allergy (e.g. allergic rhinitis) or other documented allergies, including food, contactants, and other, except for drug allergy
4. Mononeuropthy or polyneuropathy: Development of mononeuropathy, multiple mononeuropathy, or polyneuropathy (i.e. glove/stocking distribution) attributable to systemic vasculitis
5. Paranasal sinus abnormality: History of acute or chronic paranasal sinus pain, or tenderness or radiographic opacification of the paranasal sinuses
6. Extravascular eosinophils: Biopsy including artery, arteriole, or venule, showing accumulation of eosinophils in extravascular areas

For classification purpose, a patient shall be said to have Churg–Strauss syndrome if at least four of these six criteria are present

*Churg–Strauss syndrome (continued)*

small to medium-sized vessels, and associated with asthma and eosinophilia

*Microscopic polyangiitis*
No definition given by the ACR

*Microscopic polyangiitis*
Necrotizing vasculitis, with few or no immune deposits, affecting small vessels (i.e. capilliaries, venules, or arterioles). Necrotizing arteritis involving small and medium-sized arteries may be present. Necrotizing glomerulonephritis is very common. Pulmonary capillaritis often occurs

*Henoch–Schönlein purpura*

1. Slightly raised 'palpable' haemorrhagic skin lesions, not related to thrombocytopenia
2. Patients 20 years or younger at onset of first symptoms
3. Diffuse abdominal pain, worse after meals, or the diagnosis of bowel ischaemia, usually including bloody diarrhoea
4. Histological changes showing granulocytes in the wall of arterioles or venules

For purpose of classification, a patient shall be said to have Henoch–Schönlein purpura if at least two of these four criteria are present

*Henoch–Schönlein purpura*
Vasculitis, with IgA-dominant immune deposits, affecting small vessels (i.e. capillaries, venules, or arterioles). Typically involves skin, gut, and glomeruli, and is associated with arthralgias or arthritis

*Essential cryoglobulinaemic vasculitis*
No definition given by the ACR

*Essential cryoglobulinaemic vasculitis*
Vasculitis, with cryoglobulin immune deposits, affecting small vessels (i.e. capillaries, venules, or arterioles), and associated with cryoglobulins in serum. Skin and gomeruli are often involved

### Large-vessel vasculitis

#### Giant cell arteritis

GCA usually occurs in elderly persons and is the most frequent primary vasculitis. The typical clinical presentation is temporal arteritis with the characteristic temple headache (7.4). However, as occipital arteries, for example, can also be affected pain of the nuchal region or pain when combing the hair is not infrequent. Claudication of the jaw is a further frequently mentioned symptom. Due to the central retinal arteries possibly being affected, there is a high risk of vision loss, which is estimated to be over 30%. When the aortic arch or its branches are involved claudication of the arms may occur as a result of stenosis. In about 50% of cases GCA is associated with polymyalgia rheumatica, which is characterized by proximal muscle pain and often severe morning stiffness.

Histological demonstration of mononuclear infiltration with giant cells and granulomatous inflammation in a temporal artery specimen is the diagnostic gold standard (7.5). However, as this is an invasive procedure which is neither readily available nor without risk, there is an increasing practice of abandoning excision.

Duplex ultrasound might be a suitable substitute as, according to some authors, it yields a sensitivity of 82% and a specificity of 91% for the diagnosis of GCA (7.6). Recently, magnetic resonance (MR) is increasingly considered for imaging of inflamed temporal arteries. To date the available data are insufficient to assess the value of this method and the ongoing studies have to be awaited. However, for the detection of involvement of the aortic arch and its branches MRI is the method of first choice (7.7). The relevance of positron emission tomography (PET) is still under discussion. Whereas its potential value for diagnosis of large-vessel vasculitis has been demonstrated sufficiently (7.8), its use for follow-up is uncertain and there are contradictory study results.

#### Takayasu's arteritis

TA is a granulomatous inflammation of the aorta and its major branches which usually affects young women. Clinically it is characterized by constitutional symptoms such as fever, night sweats, and weight loss and later on during the course of the disease increasingly by sequelae of arterial stenosis. Symptoms of insufficient blood supply depend on the localization of the affected vessels and extend from claudication of the arms to apoplectic insult.

In addition to clinical findings, imaging studies of the blood vessels are the most important diagnostic tools. Classical angiography represents the gold standard (7.9) but is increasingly being substituted by MR techniques (7.10). Ultrasound might be helpful in discriminating

**7.4** In GCA temporal artery involvement is frequently found. Tenderness upon palpitation is a nearly pathognomonic finding. Swelling of the artery is usually not as impressive as in this patient. Pulsation might be abolished.

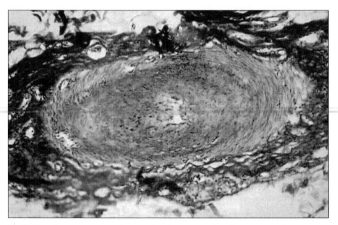

**7.5** Medium power view of a temporal artery specimen showing inflammation of the arterial wall and some multinucleated giant cells. The lumen is subtotally obstructed. (Courtesy of Prof. A.C. Feller, Dr. K. Holl-Ulrich, University of Schleswig-Holstein.)

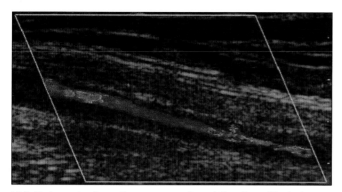

**7.6** Colour duplex ultrasonography of the A. axillaris in a patient with GCA. Besides demonstrable stenosis, the arterial wall as a sign of inflammation appears as a dark 'halo' around the lumen. (Courtesy of Prof. M. Heller, Dr. M. Both, University of Schleswig-Holstein.)

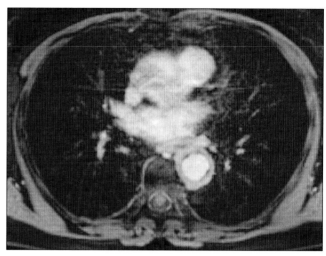

**7.7** T1-weighted MR image in a patient with GCA. The inflammation of the aorta imposes as thickening of the aortic wall and enhanced gadolinium uptake. (Courtesy of Prof. M. Heller, Dr. M. Both, University of Schleswig-Holstein.)

**7.8** Maximum intension projection of a PET of a 64-year-old patient with GCA. The symbols point to areas of increased glucose up-take as indicator of active inflammation. (Courtesy of Dr. T. Bley.)

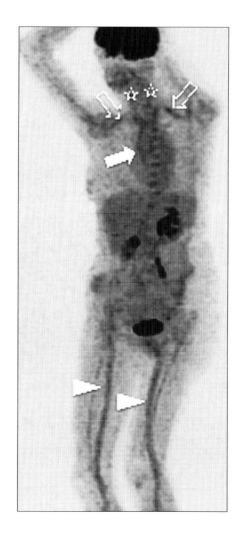

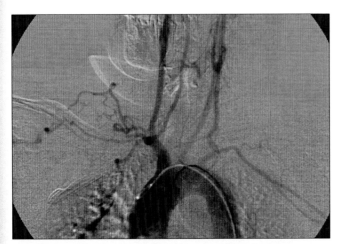

**7.9** Conventional angiography of the aortic arch in a patient with TA. An obstruction of the right subclavian artery as well as the development of collaterals can be seen. Conventional angiography is the gold standard for the detection of stenotic and aneurysmatic complications in TA and it allows immediate intervention (balloon angioplasty) if necessary. The disadvantage of this technique is its invasiveness and possible adverse events related to the use of contrast agents. (Courtesy of Prof. M. Heller, Dr. M. Both, University of Schleswig-Holstein.)

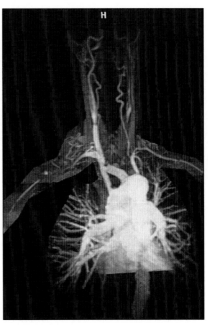

**7.10** MR angiography of the aortic arch in a patient with TA showing multiple stenotic areas. MR has the advantage of not being invasive and can image the artery wall in which oedema and uptake of gadolinium might be detectable. (Courtesy of Prof. M. Heller, Dr. M. Both, University of Schleswig-Holstein.)

between TA and arteriosclerotic lesions, e.g. in the carotid arteries. Furthermore, it might be used as a cheap and available option for follow-up (measurement of artery wall thickness). Further studies are needed to define the role of PET imaging, but as in GCA PET might be useful in determining active inflammation. Obviously histological evaluation plays no role in the diagnostic work-up of TA.

### Medium-vessel vasculitis
#### Polyarteritis nodosa

PAN is a necrotizing vasculitis affecting medium-sized or small arteries. Inflammatory microaneurysms and secondary thrombosis of the affected vessels lead to the characteristic 'pearl-necklace' aspect demonstrable in angiography (**7.11**).

Since the 1992 CHCC glomerulonephritis and vasculitis of arterioles, capillaries, or venules are excluded from the definition of PAN and if those are present MPA should be considered as a differential diagnosis. An association with hepatitis B or C virus infection has been described in up to 30% of cases. However, it is not clear if there is a causative relationship.

Besides constitutional symptoms and muscle and joint pain, the clinical presentation is determined by the distribution of the perfusion defects. Peripheral neuropathy is a common direct consequence of the vasculitis, whereas central nervous system (CNS) symptoms such as apoplectic insult are more often due to secondary hypertension and accelerated arteriosclerosis. Hypertension in PAN results from renal artery stenosis. Symptoms of the gastrointestinal (GI) tract are also common and present as temporary pain, claudicatio abdominalis, or as acute severe pain when infarction has occurred. Involvement of the coronary arteries can lead to myocardial infarction (**7.12**). Palpable nodules of skin, possibly in conjunction with livedo reticularis (**7.13**) are signs which may be detected on physical examination of the skin. The diagnosis is based on clinical and angiographic findings and, whenever available, on histological evaluation of artery biopsies. Due to changing definitions used in the last decades, classification as well as interpretation of the older literature might be especially difficult in PAN.

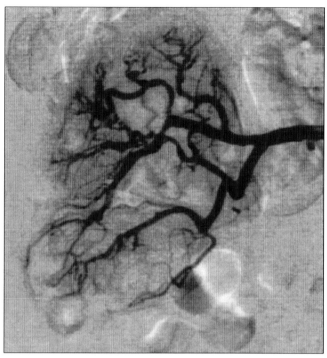

**7.11** Conventional angiography of the A. renalis in a patient with PAN demonstrating several microaneurysms. (Courtesy of Prof. M. Heller, Dr. M. Both, University of Schleswig-Holstein.)

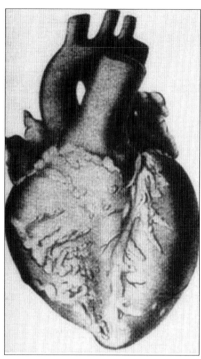

**7.12** Original illustration taken from the 1866 first description by Kussmaul and Maier. Already in this early publication the so-called 'pearl necklet' aspect of the coronary arteries was well depicted. (By permission of Mayo Foundation for Medical Education and Research. All rights reserved.)

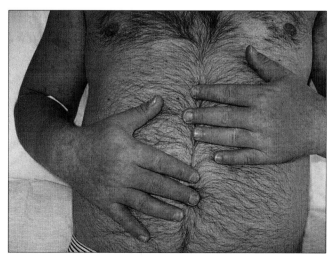

**7.13** Livedo reticularis sometimes in conjunction with palpable nodules is the main skin manifestation of PAN. Sometimes the diagnosis can be confirmed histologically from such lesions.

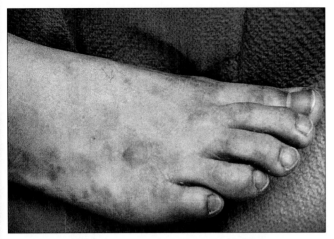

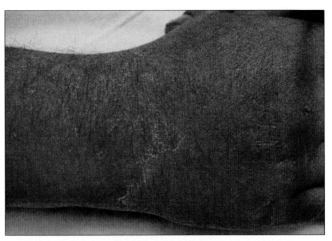

**7.14** Polymorphic exanthema in an adult with KD as well as reddening of the hands. The exanthema is not pathognomonic for this condition. Histology from the skin is nonspecific and so not recommended.

**7.15** During the course of KD, exanthema is often followed by desquamation of the skin.

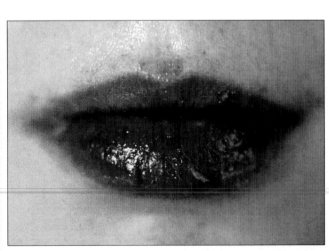

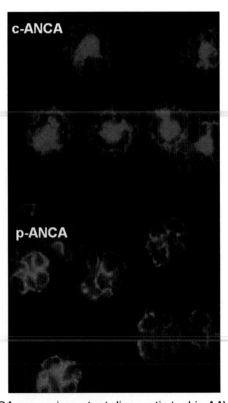

**7.16** Reddening, swelling, and erosion of the lips in a boy with KD.

**7.17** ANCA are an important diagnostic tool in AAV. Two major patterns are differentiated: the cytoplasmic pattern (upper part of the picture) and the perinuclear pattern. cANCA mostly are directed against a cytosolic protein of granulocytes, proteinase 3, whereas pANCA have a broader spectrum of possible target antigens. Most important for the diagnosis of AAV is pANCA directed against myeloperoxidase.

## Kawasaki's disease

Since patients are seldom older than 5 years KD is a domain of paediatric medicine. Patients usually present with high fever of sudden onset with or without cervical lymphadenopathy. An accompanying polymorphic exanthema might develop (**7.14**). Further skin changes such as reddening of the palms with subsequent desquamation usually accrue (**7.15**). After a few days further symptoms occur: conjunctivitis and reddening of the lips and the oral cavity with diffuse injection of the mucosa (**7.16**). A so-called 'strawberry tongue' might also be seen. Therefore KD is also known as mucocutaneus lymph node syndrome.

The most serious complication of KD is cardiac involvement with the development of inflammatory coronary artery aneurysms possibly leading to myocardial infarction (about 1% of cases). However, mild carditis might be seen in up to 50% of cases. Less frequent manifestations are: GI involvement with abdominal pain, diarrhoea and vomiting, neurological symptoms, as facial palsy or paralysis of extremities and oligoarthritis in about 20% of cases.

The most important underlying mechanism is vasculitis, especially of medium-sized arteries, which might or might not demonstrate fibrinoid necrosis. The diagnosis is mainly based on the typical combination and course of the clinical findings. Echocardiography is used to screen for possible cardiac involvement. In cases with signs of cardiac ischaemia coronary angiography might be indicated.

## Small-vessel vasculitis
### ANCA-associated vasculitides (AAV)

WG, MPA, and CSS are often referred to as AAV. Although ANCA can be found to varying degrees in all three conditions, the significant differences in pathogenesis and clinical presentation challenge the unifying concept of AAV. However, in all AAV ANCA is an important diagnostic tool (**7.17**). Whereas WG most often is associated with the cytoplasmic staining pattern in the indirect immunofluorescence assay (cANCA) and with proteinase 3 (PR3) being the target antigen, MPA and CSS are more often associated with the perinuclear staining pattern and in most cases myeloperoxidase (MPO) is identified as target antigen. *Table 7.5* presents the prevalence of ANCA in the different conditions. The classification of AAV might be challenging and in some cases inconclusive. Recently a consensus methodology for the classification of AAV and PAN has been proposed. Figure **7.18** gives an overview of the algorithm. The EUVAS has proposed definitions for different clinical stages of AAV, which should be used in the setting of therapy studies but are also useful in clinical practice (*Table 7.6*).

---

**Table 7.5 Prevalence of ANCA in different conditions according to Schönermark *et al.* (2001)**

|  | *n* | *cANCA* | *pANCA* | *PR3-ANCA* | *MPO-ANCA* |
|---|---|---|---|---|---|
| Wegener's granulomatosis | 384 | 312 | 14 | 265 | 7 |
| Microscopic polyangiitis | 40 | 1 | 26 | 0 | 19 |
| Churg–Strauss syndrome | 46 | 3 | 3 | 3 | 2 |
| Henoch–Schönlein purpura | 7 | 0 | 2 | 0 | 1 |
| Polyarteritis nodosa | 27 | 0 | 4 | 0 | 0 |
| Giant cell arteritis | 104 | 1 | 2 | 0 | 1 |
| Takayasu's arteritis | 7 | 0 | 0 | 0 | 0 |
| Systemic lupus erythematosus | 167 | 0 | 19 | 1 | 3 |
| Rheumatoid arthritis | 1412 | 0 | 121 | 0 | 1 |
| Inflammatory bowel disease | 40 | 1 | 5 | 0 | 0 |

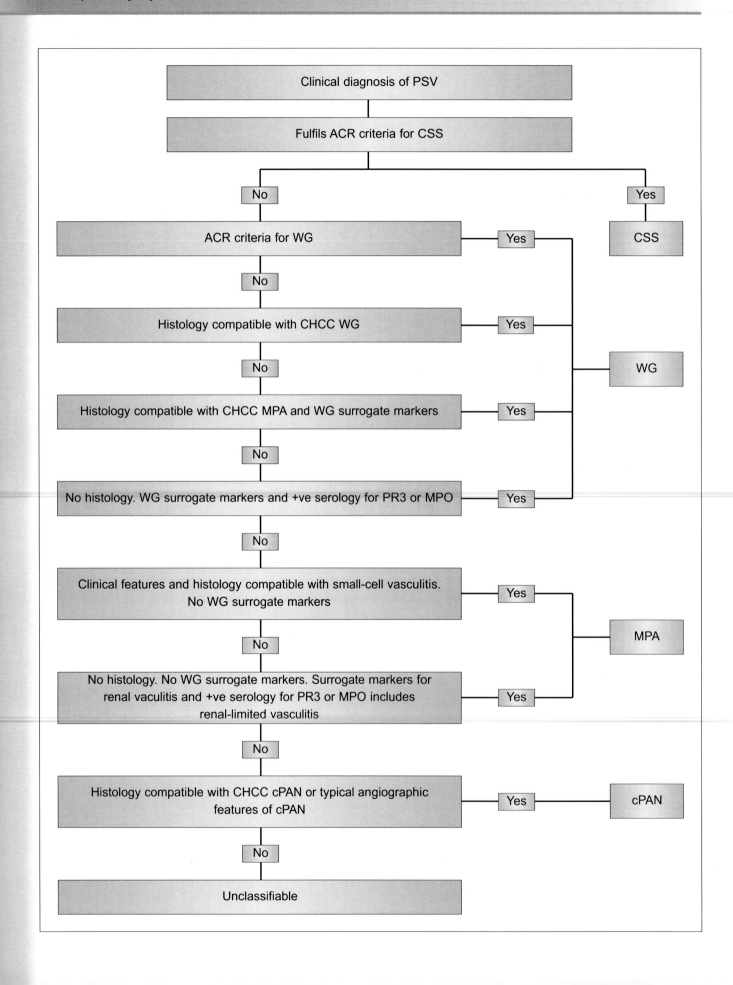

**7.18** Algorithm for the classification of primary systemic vasculitides adapted from Watts *et al.* (2007). Using this algorithm reduces the number of otherwise (according to the ACR or CHCC criteria) unclassified cases. Surrogate markers for WG refer to symptoms suggestive of granulomatous inflammation affecting the upper and lower respiratory tract. ACR: American College of Rheumatology; CHCC: Chapel Hill Consensus Conference; cPAN: classical polyarteritis nodosa; CSS: Churg–Strauss syndrome; MPA: microscopic polyangiitis; MPO: myeloperoxidase; PR3: proteinase 3; WG: Wegener's granulomatosis.

---

### Table 7.6 Definitions of activity states in vasculitis according to Hellmich *et al.* (2007)

*Remission*
Absence of disease activity attributable to active disease qualified by the need for ongoing stable maintenance immunosuppressive therapy. The term 'active disease' is not restricted to vasculitis only, but also includes other inflammatory features like granulomatous inflammation in WG or tissue eosinophilia in CSS

*Response*
50% reduction of disease activity score and absence of new manifestations

*Relapse*
Reoccurrence or new onset of disease attributable to active vasculitis
*Major:* reoccurrence or new onset of potentially organ- or life-threatening disease
*Minor:* reoccurrence or new onset which is neither potentially organ- nor life-threatening

*Refractory disease*
Unchanged or increased disease activity in acute AAV after 4 weeks of treatment with standard therapy in acute AAV, OR
Lack of response, defined as ≤ 50% reduction in the disease activity score, after 6 weeks of treatment, OR
Chronic, persistent disease defined as presence of at least one major or three minor items on the disease activity score list (e.g. Birmingham Vasculitis Activity Score [BVAS] or BVAS/WG) after ≥12 weeks of treatment

*Low activity disease state*
Persistence of minor symptoms (e.g. arthralgia, myalgia) that respond to a modest increase in the glucocorticoid (GC) dose and do not warrant an escalation of therapy beyond a modest dose increase in current medication

---

### Wegener's granulomatosis

WG usually starts as a localized infection of the upper airways characterized by granulomatous inflammation especially in the cavity of the nose. These processes might infiltrate surrounding structures like the orbitae *per continuitatem* demonstrating a somehow 'aggressive' growth (**7.19A, B**). The clinical signs are sanguinary nasal discharge, nasal deformity ('saddle nose') (**7.20**), nasal septal perforation, or proptosis (**7.21, 7.22**), eventually with eye movement disturbance. A severe complication of subglottic stenosis might occur (**7.23**). Pulmonary nodules

might be present in this stage, sometimes without clinical correlate (**7.24**).

Although WG can start as a generalized disease, more often progression from the localized state occurs after a period of time, usually several months. Generalization is characterized by the sequelae of necrotizing small-vessel vasculitis. Immediately life-threatening manifestations are rapid progressive necrotizing glomerulonephritis with crescents, alveolar haemorrhage, and as a rare complication, CNS involvement. Due to vasculitis of the

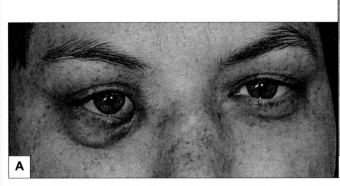
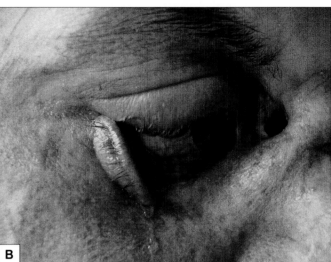

**7.19 A**: Patient with WG; **B**: despite intensive therapy destruction of the tear duct in the orbital integrity occurred due to uncontrollable granulomatous inflammation.

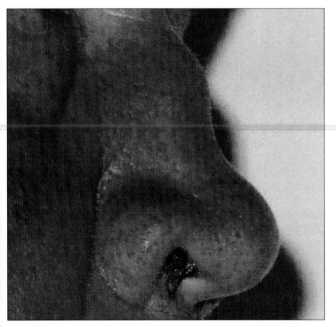

**7.20** Typical 'saddle nose' deformity and swelling in the area of the tear duct orifice due to tear duct obstruction.

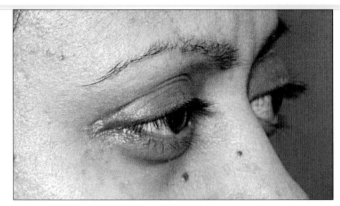

**7.21** Proptosis caused by retro-orbital granuloma masses in a patient with WG.

vasa nervorum severe disabling neuropathy, usually as mononeuritis multiplex, might occur. Glomerulonephritis usually shows no or only a few immune deposits on immunohistochemistry leading to the term 'pauci-immune' vasculitis. The incidence of affected organs at diagnosis and during follow-up is summarized in *Table 7.7*.

For the diagnostic work-up of patients with suspected WG an interdisciplinary approach involving several medical specialties is recommended. Especially, in the localized stage the ear, nose, and throat (ENT) physician is important to raise the suspicion of possible WG and to take biopsies from suspect lesions. The eye specialist, the

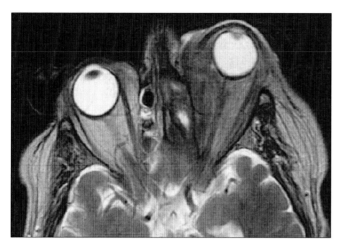

**7.22** MR image from the patient in **7.21**. Retro-orbital granulomatous inflammation leads to propulsion of the eye. (Courtesy of Prof. M. Heller, Dr. M. Both, University of Schleswig-Holstein.)

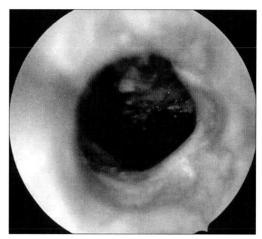

**7.23** Endoscopic view of a subglottic manifestation in WG. Stenosis might lead to severe dyspnoea and in some cases presents as an ENT emergency with the necessity of immediate intervention. (Courtesy of Prof. P. Ambrosch, Dr. M. Laudien, University of Schleswig-Holstein.)

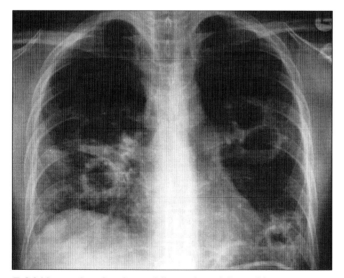

**7.24** X-ray showing large bilateral nodules with cavern formation; on the left side the development of an air-fluid level is also visible.

**Table 7.7 Involved organ systems according to Reinhold-Keller et al. (2000)**

| At diagnosis /over the whole course (%) | |
| --- | --- |
| ENT | 93/99 |
| Kidney | 54/70 |
| Lung | 55/66 |
| Eye | 40/61 |
| Heart | 13/25 |
| Peripheral nervous | 21/40 |
| CNS | 6/11 |
| Gastrointestinal | 3/6 |
| Skin | 21/33 |
| Joints | 61/77 |

neurologist, the dermatologist, the nephrologist and the rheumatologist might be necessary depending on individual clinical manifestations. Biopsies most often are taken from the inner nose. However, other organs such as skin, kidney, or nerves might also be appropriate. The specimens should be analysed by a subspecialized and experienced pathologist. For the purpose of staging, several imaging procedures are usually needed, including MRI of the head and high-resolution CT (HRCT) scan of the lungs. Further procedures, such as bronchioalveolar lavage, are used as indicated.

## Microscopic polyangiitis

MPA is the least well-defined member of the AAV group and was formally introduced into the classification of primary vasculitides in the 1992 CHCC. It is a small-vessel vasculitis which in contrast to WG shows no granulomatous component. The typical constellation is focal necrotizing crescentic glomerulonephritis in the presence of ANCA in blood, but without immune deposits in vessels or the glomerula. If ANCA is not detectable and there is no glomerulonephritis, classification might be difficult.

Constitutional symptoms are common and often precede vasculitic manifestations. Besides renal impairment, eventually presenting as rapid progressive glomerulonephritis, involvement of the lungs with (haemorrhagic) alveolitis is not uncommon and potentially life threatening (**7.25A–D**). Pulmonary fibrosis might be detectable and clinically relevant (**7.26A, B**). As in WG the skin is often affected (**7.27**). Vasculitic polyneuropathy is a further potentially disabling feature of MPA. In recent year

more 'atypical' clinical courses, e.g. with predominant neuropathy without glomerulonephritis, have been recognized. The diagnosis is mainly based on clinical features, histology, usually from renal biopsies, and the detection of ANCA. As in WG a multidisciplinary approach is recommended.

## Churg–Strauss syndrome

CSS is a granulomatous small-vessel vasculitis with marked eosinophilia as a laboratory hallmark. There are usually three disease stages: the initial stage is characterized by asthmatic complaints, polyposis, and rhinitis. In this phase of the disease CSS patients cannot be differentiated from patients who will not develop CSS. Blood eosinophilia indicates progression to the second stage in which organ manifestations such as eosinophilic pneumonia or eosinophilic gastroenteritis might develop. The different forms of the hypereosinophilic syndrome and chronic

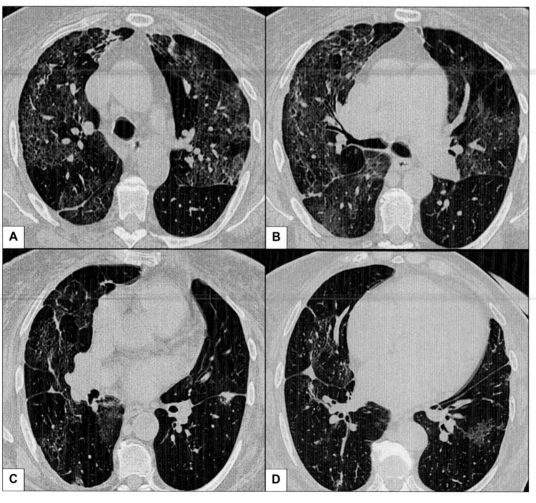

**7.25 A–D**: CT scan sections showing light glass opacities due to haemorrhage in an MPA patient. (Courtesy of Prof. M. Heller, Dr. M. Both, University of Schleswig-Holstein.)

**7.26** Pulmonary fibrosis is a not uncommon complication during the course of MPA. **A**: Conventional X-ray; **B**: corresponding CT scan sections. (Courtesy of Prof. M. Heller, Dr. M. Both, University of Schleswig-Holstein.)

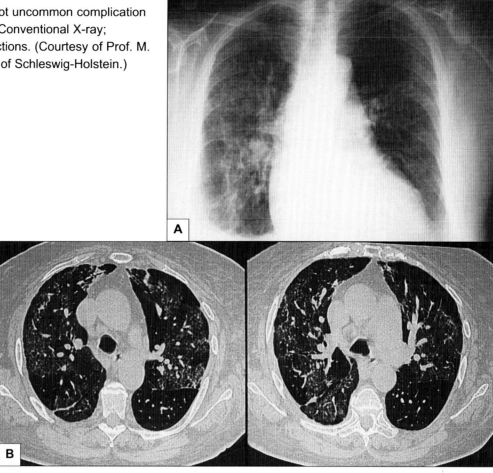

eosinophilic leukaemia, besides secondary forms of eosinophilia, are the differential diagnosis at this stage. With additional occurrence of vasculitis the stage of overt CSS is reached.

Small-vessel vasculitis often involves the skin (**7.28**), the lungs (**7.29A, B**), and the vasa nervorum (**7.30**). Severe and life-threatening manifestations include cardiac involvement, which is not uncommon and might lead to congestive heart failure, and GI inflammation with subsequent infarction.

Recent research has found differences in the clinical presentation of ANCA-positive and ANCA-negative CSS patients, with the latter being more often affected by cardiomyopathy and the former more often presenting with necrotizing glomerulonephritis. The diagnosis is strongly supported by a positive histology, i.e. the demonstration of extravascular eosinophils. For determination of the disease extent a comprehensive work-up including imaging, e.g. HRCT and muscle or heart MRI, colonoscopy, gastroscopy and bronchioscopy, neurophysiological examinations, echocardiography and so on might be necessary.

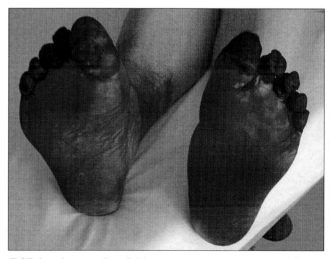

**7.27** Acral necrosis might occur as a consequence of small-vessel vasculitis. Despite immediate initiation of therapy, amputation sometimes cannot be avoided.

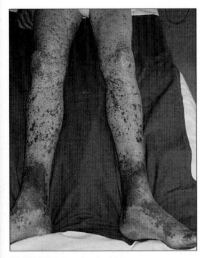

**7.28** The typical skin manifestation of AAVs is palpable purpura as depicted in this CSS patient.

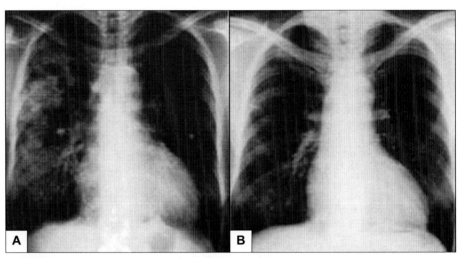

**7.29** Lung infiltrates on chest X-ray are a frequent finding in CSS. **A**: Patchy peripherally accentuated infiltrates are often the correlate of eosinophilic pneumonitis. **B**: The same patient after initiation of steroid therapy.

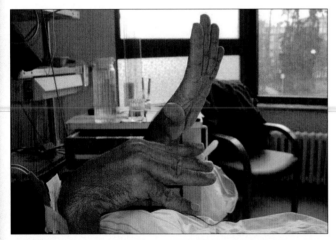

**7.30** Neurological involvement typically presents as multiple mononeuropathy. In this patient a drop hand, a sign of radial nerve impairment, has developed.

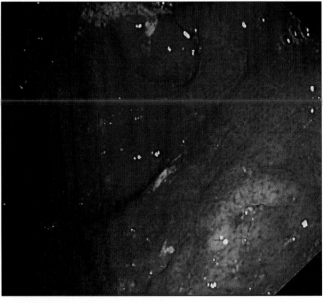

**7.31** Endoscopic view showing duodenal inflammation in a patient with HSP.

### Henoch–Schönlein purpura

HSP in contrast to the above mentioned AAV is an IgA immune complex-mediated vasculitis. The vast majority of cases affect children and the median age at onset is 6–7 years. In practically all cases there is skin involvement, typically as palpable purpura. GI symptoms are very common and the clinical spectrum reaches from mild pain and nausea to severe ischaemic pain requiring immediate surgical intervention (**7.31**). Nephritis – which usually does not present as nephrotic syndrome – occurs in about 50%

of cases. Another frequent manifestation is arthralgia/arthritis, most often of the lower extremities. Very seldom CNS symptoms or painful inflammation of the testis might present. HSP usually is self limiting and chronic disease is infrequent.

The diagnosis is mainly based on the clinical presentation. Biopsy of the skin or the kidney is usually not necessary. Endoscopic evaluation is recommended in cases of GI symptoms.

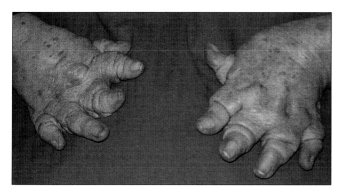

**7.32** RV usually develops in patients with long-standing severe rheumatoid arthritis as in this patient with severely destroyed finger joints.

### Essential cryoglobulinaemic vasculitis

Essential cryoglobulinaemic vasculitis (CV) is an immune complex-mediated small-vessel vasculitis. The vast majority of cases of CV are secondary to other medical conditions, most often hepatitis C virus infection. Only in cases where no underlining disease can be identified is CV classified as essential or idiopathic. Since the clinical presentation does not differ between the essential and the secondary forms, further details are given below.

### Secondary vasculitides

Secondary vasculitis develops in the context of another underlying condition. Worldwide, infectious diseases are the most common cause of vasculitis, although secondary vasculitis is often a sequela of chronic inflammatory autoimmune diseases and less frequently of neoplasia. Vasculitis due to lupus is dealt with elsewhere in this book. Here only the two most important secondary vasculitides in western countries will be delineated.

### Rheumatoid vasculitis

After long-standing severe rheumatoid factor-positive rheumatoid arthritis, rheumatoid vasculitis (RV) might develop (**7.32**) as an extra-articular complication. An overview of the frequencies of different extra-articular manifestations in rheumatoid arthritis is given in *Table 7.8*. The term RV is so far not well defined and sometimes is also used for vasculitis in the context of collagen vascular diseases.

The underlying mechanism of RV is mainly an immune complex-mediated vasculitis with or without cryoglobulins. Small vessels are principally affected but there might also be involvement of medium sized or large arteries. The clinical picture is diverse. Skin lesions are the most frequent findings (**7.33–7.35**) followed by neuropathy. Further

**Table 7.8 Frequency of extra-articular manifestations of rheumatoid arthritis according to Turesson (2003) in a series of 609 cases**

| Manifestation | n | 30-year incidence in % |
|---|---|---|
| Subcutaneous nodules | 172 | 34.0 |
| Keratoconjunctivitis | 61 | 11.6 |
| Sec. Sjögren's syndrome | 58 | 11.4 |
| Pulmonary fibrosis | 34 | 6.8 |
| Pericarditis | 21 | 5.4 |
| Pleuritis | 21 | 5.4 |
| Skin vasculitis | 19 | 3.6 |
| Others | 57 | 11.4 |

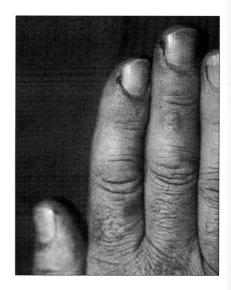

**7.33** Nailfold infarctions might be an early symptom of RV.

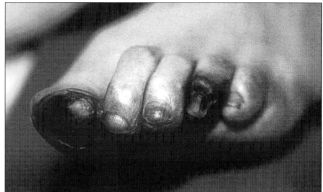

**7.34** Acral necrosis due to digital ischaemia in RV is a frequent finding and is often the first symptom.

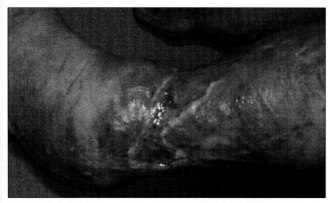

**7.35** Cutaneous ulcer is a further frequent finding in RV. It has to be differentiated from other forms of ulceration such as venous or due to arterosclerosis.

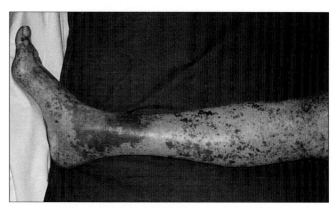

**7.36** Typical purpura in a patient with HCV. The lower extremity is preferentially affected.

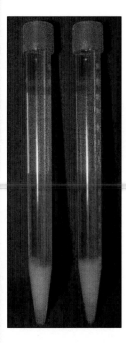

**7.37** Cryoglobulins are detected by a very simple laboratory test. Serum is separated from warm blood and kept cold for 3 days. If the test is positive, cryoglobulins can be seen as a precipitate and the amount can be measured as a cryocrit.

| Table 7.9 Conditions associated with cryoglobulinaemia |
| --- |
| **INFECTIOUS AGENTS**<br>**Viruses**<br>HIV-1, HTLV-1, HAV, HBV, HCV, adenovirus, EBV, CMV<br><br>**Bacteria**<br>Streptococcus spp., Proteus mirabilis, Brucella spp., Leptospira spp., Borrelia burgdorferi, Treponema pallidum, Chlamydia psittaci, Rickettsia conorii, Mycoplasma spp.<br><br>**Protozoa**<br>Toxoplasma gondii, Leishmania donovani, Plasmodium falciparum<br><br>**Helminths**<br>Echinococcus granulosus, Schistosoma mansoni<br><br>**Fungi**<br>Coccidioides immitis<br><br>**AUTOIMMUNE DISEASES**<br>Rheumatoid arthritis<br>Sjögren's syndrome<br>Systemic lupus erythematosus<br><br>**MALIGNANCY**<br>Multiple myeloma<br>Lymphoma, e.g. Waldenström's disease<br>Leukaemias |

manifestations might be alveolitis with subsequent fibrosis, carditis, scleritis, and colitis. The diagnosis is based on clinical findings. Histology from the skin might be useful for confirmation but usually is not necessary. Angiography can help to differentiate RV and to evaluate the extent of often associated arteriosclerosis. Other medical specialists such as the neurologist, ophthalmologist, or dermatologist should be consulted according to the clinical presentation.

### Hepatitis C-associated cryglobulinaemic vasculitis

Hepatitis C-associated cryglobulinaemic vasculitis (HCV) symptoms do not differ from symptoms of nonhepatitis-associated CV apart from the hepatitis itself. Classically Meltzer's triad comprising palpable purpura (**7.36**), arthralgia, and myalgia is seen. Acral necrosis might develop. Neuropathy can be detected in about 50% of patients, whereas glomerulonephritis is a rare complication.

Cryoglobulins are immunoglobulins that precipitate in the cold (**7.37**). According to Brouet, three types of cryoglobulin are differentiated. Type I is a single monoclonal immunoglobulin; type II is composed of a monoclonal component, usually IgM, and a poyclonal component, usually IgG; finally, type III is composed of polyclonal IgG and IgM without a monoclonal component. Recently, a type II/III has been described comprising two or more (oligo-) monoclonal components. In 80% of cases hepatitis C infection is the primary cause and is most often associated with type II cryoglobulins. Other possible underlying conditions are listed in *Table 7.9*.

In addition to the clinical presentation, laboratory tests are the cornerstone of HCV diagnosis, i.e. the detection of cryoglobulins and their differentiation, the proof of active hepatitis C virus infection by polymerase chain reaction (PCR), RF-activity, and complement consumption. Additional histology might be useful.

## Principles of management of the vasculitides

### Large-vessel vasculitides
#### Polymyalgia rheumatica and giant cell arteritis
One typical feature of polymyalgia rheumatica (PMR) is the immediate response to corticosteroid administration. Usually, 10–20 mg/day are initially effective at inducing remission. When PMR is accompanied by GCA, higher doses of corticosteroids (1 mg/kg body weight per day) are recommended. Therapy should be initiated immediately because of the risk of visual loss when the temporal artery is involved. Currently, there are no controlled data available to recommend high-dose (250–1000 mg) intravenous corticosteroid therapy (e.g. with methylprednisolone), even if visual symptoms such as amaurosis fugax or visual loss are present. However, one study found oral corticosteroids could be reduced faster after initial intravenous methylprednisolone administration. Corticosteroids should be tapered according to erythrocyte sedimentation rate (ESR)/C-reactive protein (CRP) levels and clinical symptoms to a dose of 7.5 mg prednisolone equivalent or less. Corticosteroids should be administered for at least 2 years. Aspirin should be considered as co-medication to reduce ischaemic events.

Classical immunosuppressants are used for corticosteroid sparing and in refractory conditions. Several randomized controlled studies comparing corticosteroid monotherapy to additional methotrexate (MTX) administration delivered controversial results: one study found no difference concerning relapse and corticosteroid tapering, whereas another demonstrated a reduction in both relapse frequency and corticosteroid dose in the MTX group. A meta-analysis of four studies including these two studies confirmed that MTX reduces relapse and acts as a corticosteroid-sparing agent. Azathioprine (AZA) may be an alternative for steroid sparing.

Studies assessing biological therapy in these conditions have so far been disappointing. A randomized trial with 51 PMR patients receiving either prednisone alone or prednisone and infliximab for induction did not show benefit in the infliximab group. Another study did not find infliximab used for maintenance in steroid-induced GCA effective. However, the number of patients included in these studies was small and larger studies are needed to assess the effectiveness of tumour necrosis factor (TNF) antagonists further, particularly for refractory disease. There is one case report describing successful therapy of GCA with rituximab.

Thus in many centres combination therapy with corticosteroids plus MTX or AZA is used to treat GCA when higher corticosteroid doses are needed for longer periods of time in order to avoid corticosteroid-induced side-effects (*Table 7.10*). If there are no contraindications, aspirin should be given additionally. Biological therapy cannot be recommended at this time but warrants further study.

### Takayasu's arteritis
As in GCA, steroids are used for initial therapy at a dose of 1 mg/kg/day, although no studies have been published to prove effectiveness. Immunosuppressants such as MTX and cyclophosphamide (CYC) are administered in refractory cases. An open-label pilot study with MTX demonstrated induction of remission and corticosteroid-sparing properties. CYC is often used in clinical practice for severe cases to induce remission and AZA may be used in the maintenance phase although evidence for the efficacy of CYC and AZA is weak. TNF-antagonists such as infliximab may be an option for refractory TA, as suggested by an open-label study.

### Small-vessel vasculitis
#### ANCA-associated vasculitis
WG, MPA, and CSS are summarized under the term AAV. Therapy of AAV is adapted according to disease activity and disease stage as defined by EUVAS (see *Table 7.6*): localized disease in WG refers to organ manifestation in the

### Table 7.10 Treatment of large-vessel vasculitides

| Disease | First-line treatment | For refractory disease and/or steroid-sparing properties* |
|---|---|---|
| Polymyalgia rheumatica | Corticosteroids (moderate-dose reducing) | Azathioprine<br>Methotrexate |
| Giant cell arteritis | Corticosteroids (high-dose reducing) | Methotrexate<br>Azathioprine |
| Takayasu's arteritis | Corticosteroids (high-dose reducing) | Methotrexate<br>Cyclophosphamide<br>Azathioprine<br>TNF-antagonists |

*Evidence for methotrexate in GCA only

upper and lower airways. At this stage, there is evidence from small studies that cotrimoxazole may be efficient at inducing and maintaining remission; however, even in this stage most patients will need medium or high potent immunosuppression (Holle *et al.*, 2010). Cotrimoxazole is not effective for maintenance of remission in generalized disease.

*Induction therapy for systemic disease:* For early systemic disease, MTX or CYC may be used to induce remission. In one study, remission rates did not differ significantly; however, remissions were delayed among patients suffering from extensive pulmonary involvement and who received MTX. In generalized disease or organ- and life-threatening disease, CYC and corticosteroids (for example 1 mg/kg/day orally with or without high-dose intravenous corticosteroids) are the gold standard for the induction of remission. Oral CYC (2 mg/kg body weight/day) has not yet proven to be more efficacious than pulsed CYC (15–20 mg/kg every 2–3 weeks) in the induction of remission, as shown by a meta-analysis. According to a recently published randomized controlled trial, intravenous CYC is as effective as oral CYC in inducing remission, and is associated with a lower cumulative dose and fewer adverse events; however, it is still uncertain whether intravenous CYC leads to higher relapse rates (de Groot *et al.*, 2009). In clinical practice, oral CYC often seems to be superior to intravenous CYC and is therefore preferred as the standard regimen, particularly in severe disease. In severe renal vasculitis, plasma exchange seems to be more effective at restoring renal recovery than pulsed methylprednisolone.

*Maintenance therapy for systemic disease:* Induction therapy is usually switched to maintenance therapy after 3–6 months. AZA is effective at maintaining remission compared to continued intravenous CYC, as has been demonstrated by the CYCAZAREM study. Lefluonamide and MTX may be used as an alternative for maintenance in WG but renal relapse may occur. Mycophenolate mofetil (MMF) was effective in maintaining remission in open-label trials but was inferior to AZA in a controlled randomized trial (IMPROVE). It therefore, might be seen as a 'reserve drug'.

*Biological therapy for systemic disease:* A prospective uncontrolled study with infliximab shortened the prior-to-remission period and had a steroid-sparing effect. However, the administration of etanercept additionally to CYC or MTX in a double-blind controlled trial (WGET trial) had no benefit for the induction and maintenance of remission. To conclude, the role of TNF-antagonists in AAV cannot be adequately judged from the studies performed so far. Rituximab may be a promising option for refractory AAV as shown in two small studies to date. Clinical remission was achieved in all patients and lasted as long as B cells remained undetectable. Remission was accompanied by a decrease in ANCA titre. Relapse occurred in five of 10 patients on no maintenance therapy in one study after steroids were stopped and was accompanied by a rise in ANCA titre. The protocol in these studies included four infusions of rituximab 375 mg/m$^2$ at weekly intervals. In contrast, an open trial with less frequent infusions including eight patients with refractory WG and predominant granulomatous disease found rituximab to be less effective. Two recent randomized controlled trials demonstrated non-inferiority of rituximab when compared to CYC for induction of remission in AAV. These results led to the first drug approval for AAV by the FDA. However, further studies are needed to determine the optimal indication for rituximab. According to the available data consequent substitution of CYC with rituximab in all AAV cannot be recommended. For the treatment of CSS, an open-label trial using a monoclonal IL-5 antibody showed promising results with remission induction potential (Moosig *et al.*, 2011).

## Further reading

Ball GV, Bridges SL Jr (2008). *Vasculitis*, 2nd edn. Oxford University Press, Oxford.

Cotch MF, Hoffman GS, Yerg DE, *et al.* (1996). The epidemiology of Wegener's granulomatosis. Estimates of the five-year period prevalence, annual mortality, and geographic disease distribution from population based data sources. *Arthritis Rheum* **39**:87–92.

de Groot K, Harper L, Jayne DR, *et al.* (2009). Pulse versus daily oral cyclophosphamide for induction of remission in antineutrophil cytoplasmic antibody-associated vasculitis: a randomized trial. *Ann Intern Med* **150**(10):670–80.

Fries JF, Hunder GG, Bloch DA, *et al.* (1990). The American College of Rheumatology 1990 criteria for the classification of vasculitis. Summary. *Arthritis Rheum* **22**:1135–6.

Gonzales-Gay MA, Garcia-Porrua C, Guerrero J, Rodriguez-Ledo P, *et al.* (2003). The epidemiology of the primary systemic vasculitides in northwest Spain: implications of the Chapel Hill Consensus Conference definitions. *Arthritis Rheum* **49**:388–93.

Hellmich B, Flossmann O, Gross WL, *et al.* (2007) EULAR recommendations for conducting clinical studies and/or clinical trials in systemic vasculitis: focus on anti-neutrophil cytoplasm antibody-associated vasculitis. *Ann Rheum Dis* **66**(5):605–17. Epub 2006 Dec 14.

Herlyn K, Hellmich B, Gross WL, *et al.* (2008). Stable incidence of systemic vasculitides in schleswig-holstein, Germany. *Dtsch Arztebl Int* **105**(19):355–61. Epub 2008 May 9.

Holle JU, Gross WL, Holl-Ulrich K, *et al.* (2010). Prospective long-term follow-up of patients with localised Wegener's granulomatosis: does it occur as persistent disease stage? *Ann Rheum Dis* Nov;**69**(11):1934–9. Epub 2010 May 28.

Jennette JC, Falk RJ, Andrassy K, *et al.* (1994). Nomenclature of systemic vasculitides. Proposal of an international consensus conference. *Arthritis Rheum* **37**:187–92.

Jones RB, Tervaert JW, Hauser T, *et al.* (2010). Rituximab versus cyclophosphamide in ANCA-associated renal vasculitis. *N Engl J Med* **363**(3):211–20.

Koldingsnes W, Nossent JC (2000). Epidemiology of Wegener's granulomatosis in northern Norway. *Arthritis Rheum* **43**:2481–7.

Mahr A, Guillevin L, Poissonnet M, *et al.* (2004). Prevalences of polyarteritis nodosa, microscopic polyangiitis, Wegener's granulomatosis, and Churg–Strauss syndrome in a French urban multi ethnic population in 2000: a capture-recapture estimate. *Arthritis Rheum* **51**:92–9.

Moosig F, Bremer JP, Herrmann K *et al.* Mepolizumab in refractory/relapsing Churg–Strauss syndrome. *Ann Int Med,* in press.

Reinhold-Keller E, Zeidler A, Gutfleisch J, *et al.* (2000). Giant cell arteritis is more prevalent in urban than rural populations: results of an epidemiological study of primary systrmic vasculitides in Germany. *Rheumatology* **39**:1396–402.

Reinhold-Keller E, Herlyn K, Wagner-Bastmeyer R, *et al.* (2005). Stable incidence of primary systemic vasculitides over five years: results from the German vasculitis register. *Arthritis Rheum* **53**:93–9.

Schönermarck U, Lamprecht P, Csernok E, Gross WL (2001). Prevalence and spectrum of rheumatic diseases associated with proteinase 3-antineutrophil cytoplasmic antibodies (ANCA) and myeloperoxidase-ANCA. *Rheumatology* **40**(2):178–84.

Stone JH, Merkel PA, Spiera R, *et al.* (2010). Rituximab versus cyclophosphamide for ANCA-associated vasculitis. *N Engl J Med* **363**(3):221–32.

Turesson C, O'Fallon WM, Crowson CS, *et al.* (2003). Extra-articular disease manifestations in rheumatoid arthritis: incidence trends and risk factors over 46 years. *Ann Rheum Dis* **62**(8):722–7.

Watts RA, Lane S, Bentham G, *et al.* (2000). Epidemiology of systemic vasculitis – a ten-year study in the United Kingdom. *Arthritis Rheum* **43**:414–19.

Watts R, Lane S, Hanslik T, *et al.* (2007). Development and validation of a consensus methodology for the classification of the ANCA-associated vasculitides and polyarteritis nodosa for epidemiological studies. *Ann Rheum Dis* **66**(2):222–7. Epub 2006 Aug 10.

# Index